Cataract
*Detection, measurement and management
in optometric practice*

Cataract

*Detection, measurement and management
in optometric practice*

Edited by

William A. Douthwaite PhD, MSc, FBCO, DCLP
Senior Lecturer, Department of Optometry, University of Bradford, UK

and

Mark A. Hurst PhD, BSc, FBCO
Lecturer, Department of Optometry, University of Bradford, UK

With a Foreword by Professor L.D. Pickwell

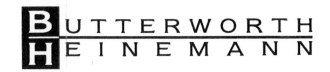

Butterworth-Heinemann Ltd
Linacre House, Jordan Hill, Oxford OX2 8DP

A member of the Reed Elsevier group

OXFORD LONDON BOSTON
MUNICH NEW DELHI SINGAPORE SYDNEY
TOKYO TORONTO WELLINGTON

First published 1993

Transferred to digital printing 2005

© Butterworth-Heinemann Ltd 1993

British Library Cataloguing in Publication Data
Cataract: Detection Measurement and
Management in Optometric Practice
  I. Douthwaite, W. A. II. Hurst, Mark A.
  617.7

ISBN 0 7506 0369 0

Library of Congress Cataloguing in Publication Data
Cataract: detection, measurement and management in optometric practice / edited by William
  A. Douthwaite and Mark A. Hurst.
  p. cm.
Includes bibliographical references and index.
ISBN 0 7506 0369 0
1. Cataract. I. Douthwaite, W. A. (William Arthur) II. Hurst,
Mark A.
[DNLM: 1. Cataract—diagnosis. 2. Cataract—physiopathology.
3. Cataract—therapy. WW 260 C35653 193]
RE451.C344 1993
617.7'42—dc20
DNLM/DLC
for Library of Congress   93-25173
                                                        CIP

Typeset by P&R Typesetters Ltd, Salisbury, Wilts
Printed and bound by Antony Rowe Ltd, Eastbourne

Contents

Contributors

William A. Douthwaite PhD, MSc, FBCO, DCLP, Senior Lecturer, Department of Optometry, University of Bradford, UK

David B. Elliott PhD, BSc, MBCO, FAAO, Research Assistant Professor, Centre for Sight Enhancement, School of Optometry, University of Waterloo, Ontario, Canada

Janet Hesler PhD, BSc, MBCO, Honorary Research Fellow, Department of Optometry, University of Bradford, UK

Mark A. Hurst PhD, BSc, FBCO, Lecturer, Department of Optometry, University of Bradford, UK

Alan H. Tunnacliffe PhD, BA, FBCO, DCLP, Dip Maths, Senior Lecturer, Department of Dispensing Optics, Bradford and Ilkley Community College, Bradford, UK

John R. Weatherill FRCS, DO, Honorary Visiting Professor, Department of Optometry, University of Bradford, UK; and Consultant Ophthalmologist, The Bradford Royal Infirmary, UK

Sally A. Young PhD, BSc, MBCO, Clinical Research Fellow, Department of Optometry, University of Bradford, UK

Foreword

This is a book for practising optometrists written by people who are not only themselves experienced practitioners but who have also extensively researched in the field of cataract. They have been working in cataract research over a period of ten years, from the beginning of what has been a new era in this field, when new methods of studying cataract have been developed. Together with two other principal centres for cataract research, they have contributed greatly to the methodology of study of lenticular opacity and its effect on vision. Recently there has been a great deal of progress in monitoring the effects of cataract on visual performance. The authors have been instrumental in this advancement of knowledge. Throughout the duration of their research they have played a major part in developing methods for assessing the progress of cataract by detecting and measuring its effect on vision and therefore its effect on the lifestyle of the patient. The necessity to use precise psychophysical methods in their research has meant that they have been at the forefront of developing and improving not only their own techniques but also in carrying out informed assessments of techniques developed by other researchers.

In this book the authors have brought together those aspects of their expertise in cataract which are of particular interest and value to practising optometrists. It provides the up to date information and relevant background material which the optometrist requires to effectively manage his/her cataract patients.

Professor L.D. Pickwell
former Head of Department of Optometry
University of Bradford

Preface

This book has been written by members of staff and researchers in the optometry department at the University of Bradford. These people have been involved in research activities associated with the monitoring of the development of cataract. The studies have been made in collaboration with the Clinical Cataract Research Unit, Nuffield Laboratory of Ophthalmology, University of Oxford, UK and the Centre for Clinical Cataract Research, Harvard Medical School, Boston, USA. During this project we became aware of the fact that many aspects of our studies were of direct interest to the practising optometrist and this provided the incentive to produce the book.

In the not too distant past, the initial detection of cataract involved a note of its presence on the record card, followed by a monitoring function at subsequent visits. Ophthalmologists advised that patients should not be referred until the fundus was becoming difficult to see, or the visual acuity was down to $\frac{6}{24}$. Patients had to suffer this significant loss of visual acuity and the quality of life was markedly reduced before any cataract operation was considered.

The current approach to the problem of cataract is completely different. The majority of patients undergo surgery at a much earlier stage in the development of the opacities. Therefore the role of the optometrist has changed to one where early detection of the condition has increased in importance. The promise of anti-cataract agents which slow down or arrest cataract development will make early detection paramount.

With this in mind, it is apparent that the optometric profession is in need of a publication which describes the optometric aspects of cataract detection and management. There is a plethora of books on cataract for the ophthalmologist but these deal with topics that are of less relevance to the practising optometrist.

This book, as the title suggests, is concerned with the detection, the quantitative monitoring and patient management by the optometrist. The introduction attempts to describe the extent of the problem both now and in the future. This is followed by a chapter on the biochemistry of the crystalline lens, which has been written assuming the reader has only a basic biochemical knowledge. Cataract is then classified into morphological types and the signs, symptoms and patient management are discussed. New techniques which hold promise as methods for quantifying the deterioration induced by the developing cataract are considered, along with techniques used to separate the influence of neural dysfunction from that produced by the cataract. A personal view of ophthalmological attitudes is described, with particular reference to current surgical techniques. The next section of the book covers the optical correction of the aphakic eye by spectacle lenses, contact lenses and intra-ocular implants.

The final chapter looks at the medical treatment of cataract by drugs and other agents. An interesting political aspect for the optometrist, is that any effective anti-cataract agent will require regular monitoring of the condition and the optometrist is in the best position to provide this service. Thus the optometrist's role in managing cataract may alter completely in the future. Indeed, if an effective agent was discovered which did not require prescribing by a medical practitioner, then the optometrist could be usefully employed in therapeutic work. This book covers the areas required to ensure that cataract monitoring, with or without therapeutic control, can be performed effectively.

W.A. Douthwaite
M.A. Hurst

1

Introduction

William A. Douthwaite

Cataract has been a major scourge of the human race with little relief except the surgeon's knife and thick spectacles until very recent times. It can be defined as a loss of transparency of the crystalline lens. It is often regarded as a lens opacity which produces a reduction in visual performance. This is a sensible rationale because of the large numbers of elderly people who have non-sight-threatening lens opacities. Often, the elderly patient is fearful of the word 'cataract' and regards the condition with considerable trepidation. One useful function that the optometrist can perform is to reassure this type of patient and to outline the great advances made in cataract surgery in recent years.

Throughout the world at least 50 million people suffer from cataract-related reduction of visual performance, with 17 million being severely disabled. In the UK, cataract is one of the four main causes of blindness. The majority of patients registered blind or partially sighted are elderly and are registered because of macular disease, glaucoma and cataract.

The cataract is dealt with by surgical intervention, followed by refractive correction using either a spectacle lens, a contact lens or an implanted intraocular lens (IOL). The trend over recent years has been towards the use of the IOL. In the past, American figures on postoperative visual acuity (VA) with IOLs have indicated that over 80% of patients up to and above the age of 80 will possess a Snellen acuity better than 6/12. It can be noted here that an acuity of 6/12 for an 80-year-old patient can be regarded as normal because of the retinal and neural degeneration associated with advancing years. Macular oedema is the main sight-threatening complication of IOL surgery, with around 5% of patients being affected. This drops to around 3% if only posterior-chamber IOLs are considered. It is likely that these figures will improve further as the techniques are refined. Ultraviolet (UV)-absorbing implants, for example, could possibly reduce the postoperative macular deterioration.

There is still a belief among patients that cataracts can only be operated on when they are mature. This is probably perpetuated by the length of the waiting lists for cataract operations. However, the point at which an ophthalmologist decides to operate is a matter of personal opinion. Patients may be treated as soon as they feel that their life style is being adversely affected and this may be when the VA is around 6/9 or better. At the other end of the spectrum patients may not be considered for surgery until the acuity is below 6/18 in the better eye.

It must be noted that some patients may be so old and frail that the operation is likely to subject them to a traumatic experience that is difficult to justify in terms of the possible visual improvement. There is also the possibility of an adverse reaction. The risks are very low but possible complications include:

- Macular oedema
- Hyphaema
- Iritis
- Corneal oedema

- IOL dislocation
- Retinal detachment
- Endophthalmitis

In some cases the expectation of improved vision is not realized or is disappointing because of some unforeseen pathology which could not be assessed before the cataract removal, the most common condition being age-related maculopathy.

There is also the possibility of the need for secondary surgical intervention. The popularity of extracapsular cataract extraction is accompanied by a concomitant increase in the requirement for posterior capsulotomies.

Half of the blindness in the world is due to cataract and this represents some 13 million people. There is a disproportionate number of cataract blind in the Third World which is not only due to a lack of medical facilities but is also due to a higher incidence rate and an earlier age of onset. Factors such as greater UV light absorption, poorer nutrition and/or a high rate of chronic diarrhoea may have some influence. Estimates of cataract blind in India are around 6 million with some $1\frac{1}{2}$ million new cases occurring each year. This inevitably means that a large number of cases go untreated and the backlog is continually rising. The situation is much the same in other parts of the Third World, for example Peru and Brazil are badly afflicted. There is also an increasing demand for cataract surgery in the developed nations. If we consider the population growth in the older age group, along with greater expectations for the quality of life after retirement, then we might estimate a considerable increase in the number of cataract operations in the next century. This may put too much strain on an already overloaded health care system. Further refinements of technique with the switch to outpatient IOL surgery may help in the short term.

It has been estimated that if the development of cataract could be delayed by 10 years, then the number of operations performed annually would decrease by some 45% as a result of patients dying before the cataract reaches a stage where it is creating visual difficulties. This is where an anticataract drug could prove most useful. If a drug were available that could stop or slow down the development of cataract, it could make a substantial contribution to combating the problem described above for both the developed nations and the Third World.

There are around 50 anticataract agents on the international market. The majority of the formulations are aimed at normalizing the lens biochemistry. The best known and most widely used agent is the Japanese formulation Catalin (also known as Clavariscan). This was developed in an attempt to inhibit the formation of a presumed group of toxic agents called quinones, which were thought to adversely affect the lens proteins. There is, as yet, no scientific evidence to show that quinones are present within the lens or the aqueous. This is typical of the drugs that are available, in that they use a therapy concept to justify their use which may be discredited as we learn more about the biochemistry of the lens. Few formulations have been clinically tested and the documented clinical trials often do not stand close inspection. Often the cataract progress was assessed using VA and refractive error only, with some studies including a slit-lamp examination and photograph. The basic problem is that we have no effective technique of objectively quantifying the development of cataract to a high degree of precision. Even if we succeed in developing suitable techniques, we must approach the problem using double-blind studies where neither the patient nor the examiner know who is using the drug and who is using the placebo. The double-blind studies that have been performed have revealed the inadequacies of the open trials that have, alas, been all too common in the investigation of anticataract drugs.

Identifying the factors that increase the risk of cataract has received a lot of attention, along with the possibility of treating cataract by drug therapy. It is hoped that these efforts will result in a reduction in the risk of being afflicted, with the possibility of preventing cataract development where the condition is detected early. The ability to quantify cataract-induced changes in visual performance has, therefore, taken on an increased importance. The optometry department in the University of Bradford has devoted considerable time and effort to developing some precise methods of quantification of changes induced by cataract. These techniques should ideally differentiate between neural and optical deterioration.

It is obviously necessary to subdivide the different types of cataract by some sort of classification system. Three major types are now recognized according to the position of the opacities in the lens. The first group is the cortical cataract of which the 'age-related' or senile cataract of the spoke variety is typical. This results from the newer lens fibres imbibing water to the extent that they eventually burst and leave opaque debris. The second group according to the morphology is the nuclear cataract which arises from an aggregation of pigmented proteins in the deeper layers of the lens. This is seen as a diffuse opacification throughout the lens nucleus. The third group is the posterior subcapsular cataract. This looks like a disc-shaped collection of patches under the posterior capsule resulting from a collection of abnormal cells. It is also possible to encounter anterior subcapsular opacities although these are comparatively rare. This neat classification system is, however, often complicated by the presence of cataract of mixed morphology in an individual eye.

There are certain factors that may predispose an eye to cataract with the most obvious being age. Exposure to the sun's rays in the more equatorial and tropical regions of the world, particularly for individuals working outside, is a probable causative factor. It is also worth noting that as the expected life span increases in the developed world, along with more outdoor recreation and holidays in exotic locations, further coupled with the depletion of the ozone layer, then lens damage by the sun's rays may develop as a problem in the more temperate latitudes. Cataract is more likely in high myopia and also in patients with glaucoma. Females are more likely to be afflicted than males. Links with cigarette smoking have been suggested. People born prematurely are probably more at risk and the premature birth rate is several times higher in the Third World than in the UK.

The treatment of cataract by drugs raises a number of questions and the one of most interest to the optometrist is what will be her or his role in this approach. In the UK, regular monitoring of incipient cataract is performed by optometrists and, when an effective drug therapy is established, there is no doubt that this role will be an even more vital part of primary vision care. The optometrist will need to concentrate her or his efforts in the direction of detecting opacities at the earliest possible time in order to maximize the potential benefits of the drug. It will, of course, be necessary to monitor the changes in the opacities with time and once again the optometrist is in the best position to provide this service. So the emphasis in the diagnosis and monitoring of cataract will be completely different from that of the present. All of this will widen the scope of optometry in vision care, and, although it is a little early for the individual practitioner to do more than monitor the progress of early cataract, optometry is undoubtedly in the forefront of research in this important field.

Lens structure, biochemistry and transparency

Mark A. Hurst

2.1 Lens structure

The lens is comprised of an avascular organ enclosed by a collagenous elastic membrane called the capsule. It is suspended by the zonular fibres and lies between the circulating aqueous and the static vitreous. The capsule's function is to support the main body of the lens, rather than to provide a barrier between it and the posterior and anterior chambers. In fact, in the young healthy eye, low molecular weight components are able to pass freely across the capsule.

Beneath the anterior capsule lies a single layer of epithelial cells. Those cells occupying the central part of the lens do not possess any mitotic activity, whereas those nearing the equatorial region of the lens do divide. These cells elongate and differentiate into fibre cells which grow from the equator in an anterior and posterior direction and constitute the lens cortex. The junctions where fibres from the opposite ends of the equator meet produce the characteristic appearance of the Y sutures. Although the lens is an ectodermal tissue, old cells are not able to be shed because they are enclosed in the capsule and the newly formed lens fibres. Instead, the oldest differentiated fibre cells are pushed deeper into the lens and lose such intracellular organelles as nuclei and mitochondria and become true mature lens fibre cells. This has consequences for both lens metabolism and transparency (see Sections 2.2 and 2.3). Thus, the size of the normal lens increases in both width [1] and weight [2] with age.

As the lens grows, its fibres are laid down in a regular manner. Nearer the nucleus of the lens some packing of the fibres takes place and results in a slight amount of dehydration of the nuclear fibre cells as compared with the younger fibres of the cortex.

2.2 Lens membranes and ionic balance

The normal lens contains about 65% water and 35% organic matter [3]. The latter comprises the cystoskeletal membranes and the structural proteins of the lens which ultimately give the lens its refractive properties.

Intracellular structural proteins can be subdivided into α-, β- and γ-crystallins and an insoluble protein fraction. Although detailed discussion of their individual properties is outside the scope of this book, an excellent review can be found in Harding [4].

The α-crystallins make up the majority. They are large molecules and therefore cannot normally pass through the membranes of the lens. In addition, they are negatively charged and together with other large charged molecules, they endow the lens with a substantial internal osmotic pressure [5]. If these internal forces were allowed their head, the net result would be an ingress of water into the lens, which would destroy the regular arrangement of the lens fibres and lead to opacity.

Fortuitously, the significant ion concentration gradients which are inherently possessed by the lens are offset, to a large extent, by the restriction of passive diffusion of ions caused by the tightly packed lens cell membranes [6]. None the less, these membranes do have a tendency to leak slightly and this allows Na^+ to diffuse into the lens and K^+ to diffuse out of it.

As a further safeguard, the lens possesses an enzyme-controlled mechanism which is able to regulate the levels of Na^+ and K^+ ions (and thereby pH), despite the slight leakage of ions through the cell membranes. The enzyme in question, Na^+,K^+-ATPase, exchanges intracellular Na^+ for extracellular K^+, thus maintaining intracellular pH by a mechanism previously described as the sodium–potassium pump.

Several studies [7,8] have shown that Na^+,K^+-ATPase is found mainly in the epithelial cell membranes. Rae and Mathias [9] outline the advantages of this location for the pump as follows:

(a) It is able to derive abundant energy for its operation in this location.
(b) It is able to transport easily into and out of the aqueous.
(c) It avoids the need to operate in the minimal extracellular spaces between adjoining packed cell fibres in the deeper cortex and nuclear regions.
(d) It avoids the need for replacement of pump molecules in a location which is not suited to protein synthesis.

Nevertheless, this gives the impression that regions distant from the anterior epithelium are deprived of the beneficial ion-regulating effects of the pump. The lens fibre cells are, however, coupled at frequent intervals along the length of adjacent membranes. These 'gap junctions' allow small molecules to pass through and permit electrical coupling of cells throughout the lens [10]. Such interconnections ensure that the active transport of the epithelial cells can pump for the cell fibres throughout the whole lens and not just for those most adjacent to the anterior epithelium.

2.3 Lens metabolism

The avascular nature of the lens emphasizes the importance of the surrounding vitreous and aqueous, since all nutrition and excretion must be serviced by these fluids. The primary purpose of all the metabolic processes of the lens is to maintain transparency. Put simply, a failure of metabolism will result in opacity.

Although the differentiating and mature lens cell fibres lack intracellular organelles which keeps both absorption and light scatter to a minimum (see Section 2.4), there are drawbacks to their absence. Firstly, DNA and RNA (normally contained in the nucleus) are not available for the repair of damaged cells. Secondly, the lack of the enzymes responsible for aerobic cellular respiration (normally stored in mitochondria) means that such cells rely on glycolysis for energy production. A consequence of this is that these cells are unable to respond promptly to demands for extra energy production. Seemingly, therefore, the central fibre cells of the normal lens are not only exposed to metabolic insult but also have a concurrent reduced ability for self-repair.

It is not surprising, then, that anaerobic glycolysis is the main metabolic pathway, by which means the lens is provided with 70% of its energy requirements [11]. Other metabolic pathways such as the citric acid cycle, oxidative phosphorylation, the hexose monophosphate shunt and the sorbitol pathway have been identified and are fully documented by Cheng and Chylack [11]. It is likely that all these pathways are under delicate control, to work in tandem and to actively interact with each other. Apart from biosynthesis, some of the energy made available by metabolism is utilized by the sodium–potassium pump.

The importance of regular lens structure via ionic balance and by sustained metabolism cannot be overemphasized. Progressive alterations in electrolyte balance do seem to occur in the majority of age-related cataractous lenses, with the shift being primarily towards increased Na^+ and Ca^{2+} and reduced K^+. It is probable that this shift in electrolyte balance causes the membrane damage seen in such lenses [12].

2.4 Theory of lens transparency

Pioneering work on corneal transparency by Maurice [13] has formed the basis of the current understanding of lens transparency, the same theory applying to both anatomical structures. The essence of his work was to show that if light impinges on a perfectly regular lattice, then diffraction takes place, albeit in such a way that the diffracted rays cancel each other out by destructive interference, allowing undiffracted rays to pass without hindrance. Thus, theoretically, light scattered from such a lattice would be zero. Goldman and Benedek [14] pointed out that in practice it is not even necessary that a regular lattic structure is involved. All that is required is that the distance between the collagen fibres in the cornea (or protein molecules in the lens) are small compared with the wavelength of light. In this case, there is considerable correlation between the phases of the light waves scattered by neighbouring fibres, and, as a consequence, any scattered light is substantially reduced. In the same study they went on to show that large amounts of scatter and therefore opacity only occur if there are considerable variations in the refractive index and if this takes place over a distance equal to, or greater than, the wavelength of light.

Of course, losses of energy do occur when light passes through the normal lens. The difference in the amount of visible light incident on the crystalline lens and that transmitted by it has been called the 'extinction' [15] and is due to both scattering and absorption of light. Ludvigh and McCarthy [16] put the loss of transmission in the order of 8% and attributed this loss to absorption. Mellerio [17], however, pointed out that it was not possible to separate transmission loss caused by absorption from that caused by scatter, and therefore it would seem that Ludvigh and McCarthy [16] actually measured the extinction. Increased amounts of extinction caused by both scattering and absorption components results in reduced transparency.

2.4.1 Scattering

The process of scattering can be subdivided into both small and large particle scatter. Small particle scatter is that which occurs from objects that are smaller than the wavelength of light, whereas large particle scatter is derived from objects several wavelengths in size [15].

Small particle scatter arises from two sources:

(a) By a vicissitude in refractive index between the low molecular weight proteins of the lens and their surroundings.
(b) By irregularities in optical anisotropy of the structure of the lens which causes birefringence.

Birefringence arises from both the macromolecular structure (form birefringence) and the overall microscopic structure of the lens (intrinsic birefringence). These two types of birefringence have opposite signs and effectively cancel each other out, so long as the structural anisotropy of the lens is maintained [18].

In the normal lens, the distance over which these fluctuations take place is small compared with the wavelength of light. Any scattering is accordingly subject to destructive interference as explained above, and little light energy is lost by this route. The fact that deeper cells and fibres are lacking in both nuclei and mitochondria contribute further to keeping small particle scatter to a minimum.

Large particle scatter takes place from the lens cell and fibre membranes. Both diffraction and reflection phenomena occur and contribute to the removal of some energy from the traversing light wave.

2.4.2 Absorption

Absorption takes place because of the presence of chromophores in the lens. Chromophores responsible for absorption of visible light are protein molecules containing tryptophan and its photo-oxidation by-products. Both radioactive and non-radioactive processes occur when light impinges on a chromophore. Fluorescent and phosphorescent emissions occur because visible light excites the chromophore which emits this radiation in an attempt to return to its ground state. Thermal and vibrational motion processes also result in dissipation of energy as molecules collide with each other.

Scatter has more effect on the optical performance of the lens than absorption. This statement can be better understood by accepting that, if a tinted spectacle lens is placed before the eye, this will certainly reduce the intensity of the optical image but not its quality. If, however, a diffusing lens is placed before the eye, the effect on intensity will be small but, because of the scatter of light, no clear image will be possible.

2.5 Mechanisms of abnormal losses of transparency

From the previous section it is apparent that transparency will be reduced by:

(a) The presence of large molecular structures which will diminish the spatial order of the regularly arranged soluble proteins. One of the major changes that take place in the molecular structure of the cataractous lens is transformation of protein molecules which creates a disturbance of the normal physical arrangement. Cataractous lenses have been found to have: reduced levels of crystallin, increased amounts of insoluble protein and increased amounts of high molecular weight protein aggregates [19]. These changes extend the distances between the protein molecules and therefore markedly increase the amount of small particle scatter. Changes in the fibre walls will lead to an increase in large particle scatter, by both a reduction of destructive interference, if the thickness increases and increased reflections if the thickness of the fibres varies.

(b) An increase in the refractive index difference between molecules and their surroundings. This would occur for example if cell walls were to break down allowing an influx of water to take place.

(c) An increase in birefringence. Any change in the basic structure of the molecular and fibre arrangement of the lens will mean that the opposite birefringences, originating from each array, no longer cancel each other out.

2.6 Normal changes in transparency with age

There is a gradual increase in the amount of light scattered by the lens with age [20–22]. The amount of back scatter accelerates as age progresses, particularly in lenses of individuals over 40 years of age [23], and is paralleled by a concomitant rise in the proportion of high molecular weight proteins, starting in the second decade of life. This scatter is thought to arise from the increased amounts of high molecular weight insoluble protein aggregates that have been converted from low molecular weight soluble proteins. Benedek [24] calculated that the molecular weight of such aggregates would need to be greater than 50 million Da in order to produce opacity, and certainly such species have been identified [25]. Biochemical analysis has revealed that normally buried

sulphydryl groups are exposed and oxidized, forming disulphide links between molecules which tie the protein chains together. Of the three types of lens protein crystallin, α, β and γ, it is the γ fraction that has the largest number of sulphydryl groups. It is therefore the most susceptible to oxidation [3]. The increase in scatter has been found to originate almost entirely from the nucleus, with only a small increase from the cortical region [26].

Scatter from the cortex is due to normal morphological variations [26], these being specular reflections [27] which increase with the natural growth of this region [28,29].

Scattering apart, an augmented amount of absorption takes place from the nucleus. This is caused by increased pigmentation and results in a change in the fluorescence and emission properties of the lens. As age progresses, the amount of fluorescent chromophores formed by photo-oxidation of tryptophan increases [30]. This has the effect of changing the wavelengths of light absorbed, causing an increasing shift towards absorption at the blue end of the spectrum and consequent yellowing of the nucleus.

Apart from the growth of the cortical region, only minor changes take place in the structure of the cortex with age, these having minimal consequences for lens transparency.

2.7 Mechanisms of cataract formation

There have been many types of experimental cataract which have been identified *in vitro* and which have been proposed as models for *in vivo* human cataracts. Since several morphological types of cataract can occur in any combination in the lens, it is possible that more than one pathway is involved. Below is a list, albeit not exhaustive, of some of the models that have been proposed.

2.7.1 Oxidation

It is conceivable that oxidation is implicated in most types of cataract and may well be the initiating event in many. Sources of potential oxidizing effects follow.

2.7.1.1 Light

Sunlight has been suggested as providing some contribution in age-related cataract development [31,32]. These theories reinforced the clinical findings of Nordmann [33] who noticed that cortical cataracts are most often seen in the inferior nasal quadrant (the position which is most exposed to sunlight). The epidemiological observations of Pirie [34] and Zigman *et al.* [35] also suggested an increased incidence of brunescent cataract in regions of the world with high levels of sunlight and in those subjects who had outdoor occupations.

Despite this evidence, Harding [4] argues strongly and convincingly that the sunlight hypothesis is unsatisfactory. In particular, he points out that the incidence of degenerative diseases such as pingeculae or pterygia, which have long been associated with sunlight, seems to have no relation to the incidence of cataract.

The wavelengths of light most likely to cause damage, however, are those between 300 and 400 nm, i.e. longwave ultraviolet (UV) light [36]. Kurzel *et al.* [37] are more specific in stating that wavelengths up to 313 nm may be effective in causing lens damage. At this wavelength, over 50% of light energy incident on the cornea is transmitted to the anterior surface of the lens [38]. When UV light of around this wavelength impinges on the lens, it is directly absorbed by one of the aromatic amino acids, tryptophan [39], which is normally present in the crystalline lens. As a result of the ensuing biochemical reaction, kynurenine is produced, which itself becomes photosensitized and forms fluorescent products and protein cross-links [40]. These cause the characteristically large insoluble coloured protein complexes found in nuclear cataract. The reaction may also produce singlet oxygen [41] which itself is a highly reactive oxidant.

2.7.1.2 Oxygen

Although this is necessary for aerobic respiration, high concentrations of oxygen in its ground state are toxic. Oxygen intermediates such as hydrogen peroxide (H_2O_2), superoxide ($O_2^\bullet$) and hydroxide ($OH^\bullet$) are even more toxic as a result of their strong oxidizing properties.

The dot in parentheses in the previous sentence indicates a molecule which has an unpaired electron – a 'radical'. Such radicals as $O_2^\bullet$ and $OH^\bullet$ are among the most potent oxidants known. They are able to decay to form a number of oxidation products and act as chain-propagating radicals in a number of auto-oxidations, including the reduction of ground state oxygen. These series of reactions result in a self-perpetuating cycle of harmful oxidative reactions.

The oxygen intermediates are formed if oxygen is reduced by donation of electrons from free radicals. Oxygen and its intermediates are responsible for the following damage to the molecular structure of the lens proteins [42].

(a) Oxidation of sulphydryl groups by oxygen in its ground state giving rise to protein-to-protein disulphide bonds and hence conversion from soluble to insoluble proteins.

(b) Oxidation of the amino acids cysteine and methionine by H_2O_2. This results in the formation of disulphide bonds and sulphoxide respectively. Sulphoxide is associated with insoluble yellow and brown proteins.

2.7.2 Failure of protective mechanisms

As will be appreciated from the preceding text, the consequences of damage caused by unchecked oxidative reactions are far reaching. Within a short space of time, the crystalline lens would become cataractous. Fortunately, the potentially damaging effects of oxygen are reduced by an in-built system of defence mechanisms, aimed at giving both general protection against a number of oxidants and also at specific oxidizing agents. Quantitatively, glutathione is the most notable. Reduced levels of glutathione have been correlated with the occurrence of cortical lens opacities. Glutathione prevents the formation of the disulphide bonds and hence the conglomeration of high molecular weight protein aggregates found in denatured lens protein [43]. Detoxification of H_2O_2 is carried out by a number of enzyme systems which are derived from glutathione. H_2O_2 is in relatively high concentration in the aqueous of cataractous lenses [44] and has not only been shown to react with cysteine and methionine but also has a markedly deleterious effect on the sodium–potassium pump system of the anterior epithelium [45]. Failure of the pump has been linked with both cortical cataracts [46] and posterior subcapsular cataracts [47]. Catalase is another enzyme which, although unrelated to glutathione, is also capable of decomposing

H_2O_2. Superoxide dismustase (SOD) has been demonstrated to exist in the lens and, in particular, in the anterior epithelium. It has the function of scavenging $O_2^{\bullet}$, thereby converting it to H_2O_2 and oxygen, which can be dealt with in turn by glutathione and catalase. Reduced activity of SOD has been noted in both nuclear and cortical cataracts [48].

Antioxidants such as ascorbic acid (vitamin C) and α-tocopherol (vitamin E) are capable of scavenging $O_2^{\bullet}$, thereby interrupting oxidative chain reactions and hence reducing the net oxidative damage [49].

The presence of pigments in the lens which may have occurred as a result of photo-oxidation, nevertheless reduces the amount of light which can cause further damage.

2.7.3 Raised blood sugar levels

The cataracts formed by excess sugar (sugar cataracts) are the only type for which a single mechanism has been identified. This is the variety that occurs in the diabetic patient whose blood sugar levels are poorly controlled. 'Sugar cataracts' are caused by the conversion of surplus sugar to sugar alcohol by the enzyme aldose reductase. These sugar alcohols accumulate in the epithelium and the lens fibres and render the intracellular contents hypertonic relative to the extracellular spaces. This osmotic imbalance results in a net ingress of water into the cells, causing swelling and localized changes in refractive index and hence opacity. Aldose reductase is found in highest concentration in the anterior epithelium and superficial cortical fibres [50], and this may account for the localized cortical and posterior subcapsular opacities which are characteristic of diabetic cataracts.

As intimated earlier, excess sugar is most likely to occur in the diabetic. In this case the cataract would not be recognized as an age-related idiopathic type. Chylack [51], however, has inferred that rather than a high blood sugar level being the initiating event, it may be variation in blood sugar that causes the disruption of the lens epithelium and fibres. van Heyningen [52] has claimed that cataract may be more prevalent in non-diabetics who have elevated blood sugar levels. The question to be answered is this: is it possible for elevated and variable blood sugar levels to occur in the non-diabetic patient? If this were to occur, the

cataracts would presumably be formed in a similar way to the above mechanism.

2.7.4 Abnormal calcium levels

It has been apparent for some time that Ca^{2+} has a role to play in the formation of cataract. Adams [53] noticed that cataract patients had a higher than normal plasma Ca^{2+} concentration. Ireland [54] reported cataract development in a significant number of patients made hypocalcaemic by surgical removal of the parathyroid, and Duncan and Jacob [55] reported high Ca^{2+} levels in human cataractous lenses.

Extrusion of Ca^{2+} is carried out in the lens by the enzyme Ca^{2+}-ATPase. The activity of this enzyme in the epithelium is 30 times that of the enzyme in the nucleus. It has been found by Hightower and Reddy [56] that, as the severity of a nuclear cataract increases, so does the amount of bound Ca^{2+}. Fagerholm [57] exposed lenses to Ca^{2+} at a concentration normally found in the aqueous and observed that subcapsular opacities were formed.

Hypocalcaemia causes a disruption of the normal Na^+ and K^+ gradients in the lens. This not only allows an osmotic imbalance to take effect but, according to Shinohara and Piatigorsky [58], also inhibits protein synthesis. This would have the greatest effect on the fibres at the posterior subcapsular region of the lens, since this is the furthest away from the lens epithelium and therefore least amenable to repair.

2.7.5 Diarrhoea

Diarrhoea is considered by Harding [59] to be a possible cause of nuclear cataract. Harding's work has been supported, albeit in an epidemiological study, by Minassian *et al.* [60] who claimed a 21 times increased risk of cataract in patients who had been exposed to two cholera-like episodes of diarrhoeal disease. Harding's theory regarding the possible diarrhoeal mechanism is based on the systemic effects of diarrhoeal syndrome, which are at least four-fold:

(a) Malabsorption of nutrients leading to malnutrition. This has been recognized as a risk factor in cataract formation.
(b) Reduction of blood pH. This has been found to cause *in vitro* cataract of the mouse lens [61].

(c) Plasma fluctuations of electrolyte concentration and hence dehydration. Although the dehydration produced after one event of diarrhoea would be unlikely to cause cataract, numerous episodes would produce cycles of osmotic imbalance. If this occurs over a period of years, it is not inconceivable that lens opacities would be formed in a similar way to that which occurs in the diabetic.

(d) Increased levels of blood urea. Similar osmotic imbalances occur to those above. In addition, it is possible that urea could equilibrate with cyanate which can chemically bind to the lens proteins, reduce levels of glutathione and affect lens transport and metabolic systems [62].

In 1987, Harding and van Heyningen [63] published the results of an epidemiological study of cataract in the city of Oxford, in an attempt to identify some of the risk factors associated with the disease. Amongst other findings, they found that diarrhoea was a significant risk factor even in Oxford.

2.7.6 Phase separation opacification

This pathway to opacification is normally demonstrated by lowering the temperature surrounding an extracted experimental lens [64]. It has also been demonstrated *in vivo* in the rat fed on a diet of galactose (acting as an animal model for diabetic cataract). It usually takes the form of a nuclear or perinuclear opacity which disappears as the temperature is raised. The phenomenon is due to separation of the lens cell cytoplasm into two or more parts, each of which has different protein concentrations [33]. Substances such as H_2O_2 and cyanate (see Sections 2.7.1 and 2.7.5) raise the temperature at which phase separation takes place, while glutathione (see Section 2.7.2) decreases it. This has encouraged the view that phase separation may play a role in human cataract formation.

2.7.7 Mechanical Stress

The question as to whether mechanical stress could be capable of causing cataract was first raised by Pau [65] who suggested, albeit from clinical observation, that accommodative stress could cause lens opacification. Fisher [66] took this postulation a stage further by inducing mechanical stress on excised human lenses. This was achieved by rotating the lenses to induce radial stress of a similar type to that which would occur *in vivo* by the process of accommodation. He found that the stresses so produced resulted in an opacification of the tested lenses which resembled that of cortical cataract. Fisher [66] concluded that the combined effects of the lack of elasticity of the capsule and the rigidity of the nucleus resulted in most of the energy produced by excessive accommodative effort being dissipated almost entirely within the substance of the lens. This could result in excessive movement of the lens fibre junctions and hence layers of optical discontinuity and opacity.

References

1. Brown, N. Dating the onset of cataract. *Transactions of the Ophthalmological Society of the U.K.,* **96**, 18–20 (1976)
2. Harding, J.J., Rixon, K.C. and Marriott, F.H.C. Men have heavier lenses than women of the same age. *Experimental Eye Research,* **25**, 651 (1977)
3. Lerman, S. Lens transparency and ageing. In *Ageing of the Lens* (edited by F. Regnault, O. Hockwin and Y. Courtois), Elsevier, Amsterdam, pp. 263–279 (1979)
4. Harding, J. *Cataract. Biochemistry, Epidemiology and Pharmacology,* Chapman and Hall, London (1991)
5. Patmore, L. and Duncan, G. The physiology of lens membranes. In *Mechanisms of Cataract Formation in the Human Lens* (edited by G. Duncan), Academic Press, London, pp 193–217 (1981)
6. Paterson, C.A., Delamere, N.A. and Holmes, D.L. Calcium and lens membrane permeability characteristics. In *Ageing of the Lens* (edited by F. Regnault, O. Hockwin and Y. Courtois), Elsevier, Amsterdam, pp. 121–130 (1979)
7. Bonting, S.L., Caravoggio, L.L. and Hawkins, N.M. Studies on Na-K activated ATPase. VI. Its role in cation transport in the lens of cat, calf and rabbit. *Archives of Biochemistry,* **101**, 47–55 (1963)
8. Palva, M. and Palkama, A. Sodium-potassium activated adenosine triphosphatase activity in the rat lens. A histochemical and biochemical study. *Acta Ophthalmologica (Suppl)(Kbh),* **123**, 82–87 (1974)
9. Rae, J.L. and Mathias, R.T. The physiology of the lens. In *The Ocular Lens* (edited by H. Maisel), Marcel Dekker Inc., New York, pp. 93–121 (1984)
10. Kusak, J., Maisel, H. and Harding, C.V. Gap junctions of chick lens fibre cells. *Experimental Eye Research,* **27**, 495–498 (1978)

11. Cheng, H.M. and Chylack, L.T. Lens metabolism. In *The Ocular Lens* (edited by H. Maisel), Marcel Dekker Inc., New York, pp. 223–264 (1984)

12. Gandolfi, S.A., Melli, E, Tomba, M.C. and Maraini, G. Membrane damage in human senile cataract. Evidence from radiotracer fluxes and measurement. In *The Lens: Transparency and Cataract* (edited by G. Duncan), Eurage, Rijswijk, pp. 97–102 (1986)

13. Maurice, D.M. The structure and transparency of the cornea. *Journal of Physiology*, **136**, 263–286 (1957)

14. Goldman, J.N. and Benedek, G.B. The relationship between morphology and transparency of the non-swelling stroma of the shark. *Investigative Ophthalmology*, **6**, 574–600 (1967)

15. Trokel, S. The physical basis for the transparency of the crystalline lens. *Investigative Ophthalmology*, **1**, 493–501 (1962)

16. Ludvich, E. and McCarthy, E.F. Absorption of visible light by the refractive media of the eye. *Archives of Ophthalmology*, 37–51 (1938)

17. Mellerio, J. Light absorption and scatter in the human lens. *Vision Research*, **11**, 129–141 (1971)

18. Bettleheim, F.A. On the optical anisotropy of the lens fiber cells. *Experimental Eye Research*, **21**, 231–234 (1975)

19. Harding, J.J. Changes in lens proteins in cataract. In *Molecular and Cell Biology of the Eye Lens* (edited by H. Bloemendal), Wiley, New York, pp. 327–366 (1981)

20. Wolf E. Glare and age. *Archives of Ophthalmology*, **64**, 502–514 (1960)

21. Goldmann, H. Senile changes of the lens and vitreous. *American Journal of Ophthalmology*, **57**, 1–13 (1964)

22. Elliott, D.B. and Hurst, M.A. Assessing the effect of cataract: A clinical evaluation of the Opacity Lensmeter 701. *Optometry and Visual Science*, **66**, 257–263 (1989)

23. Zeimer, R.C. and Noth, J.M. A new method of measuring in-vivo, and study of lens scatter, fluorescence and transmittance. *Ophthalmic Research*, **16**, 246–255 (1984)

24. Benedek, G.B. Theory of the transparency of the eye. *Applied Optics*, **10**, 459–473 (1971)

25. Jedziniak, J.A., Kinoshita, J.H., Yates, E.M., Hocker, L.O. and Benedek, G.B. On the presence and mechanism of formation of heavy molecular weight aggregates in human normal and cataractous human lenses. *Experimental Eye Research*, **15**, 185–192 (1973)

26. Spector, A., Li, S. and Sigelman, J. Age-dependant changes in the molecular size of human lens proteins and their relationship to light scatter. *Investigative Ophthalmology and Visual Science*, **13**, 795–798 (1974)

27. Weale, R.A. Real light scatter in the human crystalline lens. *Graefes Archives for Clinical and Experimental Ophthalmology*, **224**, 463–466 (1986)

28. Sigelman, J., Trokel, S.L. and Spector, A. Quantitative biomicroscopy of lens light back scatter. *Archives of Ophthalmology*, **92**, 437–442 (1974)

29. Mellerio, J. Yellowing of the human lens: Nuclear and cortical contributions. *Vision Research*, **27**, 1581–1587 (1987)

30. Lerman, S. Chemical and physical properties of the normal and ageing lens: spectroscopic (UV, fluorescence, phosphorescence and NMR) analyses. *American Journal of Optometry and Physiological Optics*, **64**, 11–62 (1987)

31. Hiller, R., Giacometti, L. and Yuen, K. Sunlight and cataract: An epidemiologic investigation. *American Journal of Epidemiology*, **105**, 450–459 (1977)

32. Taylor, H.R. The environment and the lens. *British Journal of Ophthalmology*, **64**, 303–310, (1980)

33. Nordmann, J. Problems in cataract research. *Ophthalmic Research*, **3**, 323–359 (1972)

34. Pirie, A. Photo-oxidation of proteins and comparison of photo-oxidised proteins with those of the cataractous human lens. *Israel Journal of Medical Science*, **8**, 1567–1573 (1972)

35. Zigman, S., Datiles, M. and Torczynski, E. Sunlight and human cataracts. *Investigative Ophthalmology and Visual Science*, **18**, 462–467 (1979)

36. Chylack, L.T. Mechanisms of senile cataract formation. *Ophthalmology*, **91**, 596–602 (1984)

37. Kurzel, R., Myron, L., Wolbarsh, T. and Yamanashi B. UV radiation effects on the human eye. *Photochemistry and Photobiology Reviews*, **2**, 133–167 (1977)

38. Kinsey, V.E. Spectral transmission of the eye to ultraviolet radiations. *Archives of Ophthalmology*, **39**, 508–513 (1948)

39. Borkman, R.F. Cataracts and photochemical damage in the lens. In *Human Cataract Formation; Ciba Foundation Symposium* **106**, Pitman, London, pp. 88–99 (1984)

40. Fujimori, F. Crosslinking and blue fluorescence of photooxidized calf lens alpha-crystallin. *Experimental Eye Research*, **34**, 381–387 (1982)

41. Walrant, P. and Santus, R. N-formyl-kynurenine, a tryptophan photo-oxidation product, as a photo-dynamic sensitizer. *Photochemistry and Photobiology*, **19**, 411–417 (1974)

42. Augusteyn, R.C. Protein modification in cataract: Possible oxidative mechanisms. In *Mechanisms of Cataract Formation in the Human Lens* (edited by G. Duncan), Academic press, London, pp. 71–116 (1981)

43. Reddy, V.N and Giblin, F.J. Metabolism and function of glutathione in the lens. In *Human Cataract Formation; Ciba Foundation Symposium* **106**, Pitman, London, pp. 65–87 (1984)

44. Spector, A. and Garner, W.H. Hydrogen peroxide and human cataract. *Experimental Eye Research*, **33**, 673–681 (1981)

45. Garner, W.H, Garner, M.H, and Spector, A. H_2O_2-induced uncoupling of bovine lens Na^+, K^+-ATPase. *Proceedings of the National Academy of Sciences of the United States of America*, **80**, 2044–2048 (1983)

46. Spector, A. The search for a solution to senile

cataracts. *Investigative Ophthalmology and Visual Science*, **25**, 130–146 (1984)

47. Phillipson, B.T. and Fagerholm, P.P. Lens changes responsible for light scattering in some types of senile cataract. In *The Human Lens in Relation to Cataract; Ciba Foundation Symposium* **19**, Elsevier, London, pp. 45–58 (1973)

48. Augestyn, R.C. Protein modification in cataract: Possible oxidative mechanisms. In *Mechanisms of Cataract Formation in the Human Lens* (edited by G. Duncan), Academic Press, London, pp. 71–116 (1981)

49. Fridovich, I. Oxygen: aspects of its toxicity and elements of defence. In *Proceedings of the First International Symposium on the Light and Oxygen Effects on the Eye* (edited by S.D. Varma and S. Lerman), IRL Press, Oxford, pp. 1–2 (1984)

50. Akagi, Y., Yajima, Y., Kador, P.F., Kuwabara, T. and Kinoshita, J.H. Localization of aldose reductase in the human eye. *Diabetes*, **6**, 562–566 (1984)

51. Chylack, L.T. Sugar cataracts – possibly the beginning of medical anti-cataract therapy. In *Mechanisms of Cataract Formation in the Human Lens* (edited by G. Duncan), Academic press, London, pp. 237–252 (1981)

52. van Heyningen, R. What happens to the human lens in cataract? *Scientific American*, **233**, 70–83 (1975)

53. Adams, D.R. The role of calcium in senile cataract. *Biochemical Journal*, **23**, 902–912 (1929)

54. Ireland, A.W., Hornbrook, J.W., Neale, F.C. and Posen, S. The crystalline lens in chronic surgical hypoparathyroidism. *Archives of Internal Medicine*, **122**, 408–411 (1968)

55. Duncan, G. and Jacob, T.J.C. The lens as a physicochemical system. In *The Eye* (edited by H. Davson), Academic Press, London, vol 1B, pp. 159–206 (1984)

56. Hightower, K.R. and Reddy, V.N. Calcium content and distribution in human cataract. *Experimental Eye Research*, **34**, 413–421 (1982)

57. Fagerholm, P.P. The influence of calcium on lens fibres. *Experimental Eye Research*, **28**, 111–112 (1979)

58. Shinohara, T. and Piatigorsky, J. Regulation of protein synthesis, intracellular electrolytes and cataract formation *in vitro*. *Nature*, **270**, 406–411 (1977)

59. Harding, J.J. Changes in lens proteins in cataract. In *Molecular and Cell Biology of the Eye Lens* (edited by H. Bloemendal), Wiley, New York, pp. 327–366 (1981)

60. Minnassian, J. General discussion. In *Human Cataract Formation; Ciba Foundation Symposium* **106**, Pitman, London, pp. 40–47 (1984)

61. Weinstock, M. and Scott, J.D. Effect of various agents on drug-induced opacities of the lens. *Experimental Eye Research*, **6**, 368–375 (1967)

62. Harding, J.J. and Rixon, K.C. Carbamylation of lens proteins: a possible risk factor in cataractogenesis in some tropical countries. *Experimental Eye Research*, **31**, 567–571 (1980)

63. Harding, J.J. and van Heyningen, R. Epidemiology and risk factors for cataract. *Eye*, **1**, 537–541 (1987)

64. Tardieu, A. and Delaye, M. Eye lens transparency analysed by X-ray and light scattering. In *The Lens: Transparency and Cataract* (edited by G. Duncan), Eurage, Rijswijk, pp. 49–56 (1986)

65. Pau, H. Article on the genesis of cataract. *Archives of Ophthalmology*, **150**, 340–357 (1950)

66. Fisher, R.F. Human lens fibre transparency and mechanical stress. *Experimental Eye Research*, **16**, 41–49 (1973)

Age-related and other cataract morphologies

Sally A. Young

3.1 Introduction

Although the vast majority of cataracts encountered in clinical practice are age-related in origin, the optometrist does come across other cataract types. The following discussion has been limited to those opacities that occur with some frequency in practice and generally disrupt central visual acuity (VA). In most cases, these cataracts are congenital (Sections 3.2–3.4), metabolic (Sections 3.6–3.9), or secondary to cataractogenic stresses (Section 3.10) such as radiation, trauma and local eye disease.

3.2 Congenital cataract

Some 14% of all cases of childhood blindness are caused by congenital cataract [1]. In most cases, congenital cataracts are stationary, occurring bilaterally and are associated with little or no visual disability. The patient may develop normal VA despite the presence of a lens opacity [2]. In fact, many congenital cataracts are not diagnosed until late in life, because of the lack of any signs or symptoms indicative of their presence [3]. Developmental remnants of the vascular network that surround the lens in foetal life (persistent pupillary membrane or Mittendorf's dot, for example) occur with great frequency and rarely interfere with VA [4].

Congenital cataracts may be either genetic or non-genetic and are often associated with other ocular or systemic abnormalities. When treatment is required, the need for early surgical intervention (before 2–3 months of age) has been emphasized [5]. This is the critical period for the development of a fixation reflex [6,7].

Congenital cataracts occur as an isolated hereditary finding in about 20% of cases and usually have an autosomal dominant transmission [8]. Maternal disease (especially rubella infection or endocrine disturbance) accounts for a further 20% of cases [8]. Congenital cataracts are frequently associated with low birth weight for age and central nervous system abnormalities, such as mental retardation, convulsions or cerebral palsy. Approximately 6% of congenital cataracts are associated with other ocular anomalies, such as aniridia and coloboma [8]. A very large proportion of congenital cataracts, between 35% and 50%, are therefore sporadic and of unknown aetiology [1].

3.3 Congenital cataract morphologies

The four main types of congenital cataract morphology are described below.

3.3.1 Zonular/lamellar cataract

Zonular cataracts are the most common type of congenital cataract, accounting for about 50% of the total [9]. The cataracts are usually bilateral, the degree of visual loss varying with the diameter and density of the affected lamella.

The opacity is acquired when the developing lens fibres are affected by a cataractogenic stimulus, a common cause being galactosaemia [9], for a limited period of time. The opacity affects one lamella so that it encircles the lens both anteriorly and posteriorly, forming an apparently hollow disc. The zone of opacification is surrounded on either side by clear lens. A second lamella is often subsequently affected to a lesser extent, forming a delicate envelope surrounding the main opacity. The location of the opacity varies with the time of formation, in most cases occurring in the outer foetal nucleus or inner adult nucleus [4].

Zonular cataract may be invisible at birth or develop in infancy or adolescence. This gives rise in adolescence to a large more peripheral opacity, with greater visual impairment.

Other features of the cataract include the presence of anterior and posterior riders. These are spoke-like opacities in the outer lamellae extending from the equator towards the centre of the lens. Riders tend not to occur when the causative factor has ceased abruptly [9].

3.3.2 Polar cataracts

Polar cataracts involve both the capsule and the underlying layers of the cortex. Cataracts are usually bilateral and disc-shaped but may present in a variety of shapes or positions. They occur at either the anterior or posterior pole of the crystalline lens. At the anterior pole, the opacity may be associated with a persistent pupillary membrane or with a corneal opacity. The most common cause of posterior polar cataract is a persistent hyaloid artery remnant [9].

Polar opacities are usually congenital but can also be the result of trauma (Section 3.10.3), particularly minor penetrating injuries from which the capsule has healed with scarring [9]. Visual loss resulting from polar cataract varies with its size, density and position within the pupillary area. The majority of polar cataracts do not significantly affect central VA, however and so do not require surgical intervention [4].

3.3.3 Sutural or stellate cataracts

Sutural cataracts involve the anterior or posterior Y sutures of the crystalline lens. Sutures may be involved asymmetrically, so that one or two branches of the Y are involved, or one arm is longer than the other. The Y sutures are formed earlier than any others, representing the line of intersection of the primary lens fibres and forming the anterior and posterior borders of the embryonic nucleus. Most sutural cataracts occur at this level. Opacities are usually, therefore, congenital, static and bilateral and have minimal effect on VA [9].

Approximately 3% of all premature babies develop transient opacities in the apices of the posterior Y sutures during the first 2 weeks after birth [10]. Although these transient opacities can progress to complete vacuolar opacification of the posterior subcapsular area, regression is usually complete by 25 days from the onset [9].

3.3.4 Embryonal nuclear cataract

This opacity affects only the primary lens fibres and is confined to the embryonic nucleus, the lens having no cortex at birth. The opacity is therefore spherical or ovoid, static and frequently bilateral [4]. The foetal nucleus is occupied by small discrete white dots, with the central clear interval varying in involvement. Central VA is usually affected slightly.

3.4 Congenital cataracts associated with recognized systemic conditions

Congenital cataract can be due to a number of disease processes and the most frequently encountered are listed below.

3.4.1 Rubella cataract

Rubella is the most important cause of total congenital cataract, accounting for 20% of all congenital cataracts in one series [8]. It results from foetal infection by the rubella virus during the first trimester of pregnancy. If the mother is infected during this period, there is a 50% chance [9] that the infant will develop the classic triad of the congenital rubella syndrome (eye, ear and heart defects [11]). Prevention of rubella through vaccination probably offers the safest and most effective method of reducing the incidence of the disease [12].

The virus is known to inhibit mitosis and cell division in many foetal tissues. Involvement of the lens vesicle, at the time of elongation of the posterior epithelial cells, leads to the abnormal lens development. Rubella cataract typically presents as a slightly eccentric dense white core opacity, with lesser opacification of the surrounding cortex. A total cataract may develop with time. Other ocular manifestations of the disease include pigmentary retinopathy, strabismus, microphthalmia and iritis. Pupillary dilation is frequently incomplete because of the involvement of dilator fibres [9]. Early referral to an ophthalmologist will optimize the chances of successful cataract extraction. Aspiration surgery is frequently difficult because of poor pupillary dilation, a shallow anterior chamber and microphthalmia [12]. Better results may be obtainable by pars plicata lensectomy and vitrectomy with an automated vitrectomy instrument [9].

3.4.2 Galactosaemia

This disease is due to an autosomal recessive deficiency of galactose-1-phosphate uridyltransferase, the enzyme that converts galactose 1-phosphate to uridine diphosphogalactose. The disease is manifest in patients given milk products that contain the disaccharide, lactose (glucose plus galactose). In the presence of lactose, the enzyme deficiency leads to the accumulation of galactose 1-phosphate and galactose. Galactose is converted by the enzyme aldose reductase (AR) to the sugar alcohol, galactitol. The accumulation of galactitol within lens cells creates a hypertonic state, which is neutralized by the influx of water. The entry of water leads to swelling, membrane disruption and opacification of the lens [13].

Cataracts are not apparent at birth but usually develop within the first few months. A central nuclear opacity appears, which may progress to opacification of the foetal nucleus [12], although cataracts can be reversed in their early stages by a galactose-free diet [14].

Severe systemic manifestations of the disease include mental retardation, growth inhibition and hepatic dysfunction.

3.4.3 Galactokinase deficiency

This is due to an autosomal recessively inherited deficiency of the enzyme galactokinase, the enzyme that converts galactose to galactose 1-phosphate. Lack of this enzyme leads to the accumulation of galactose, which is then converted into galactitol [12]. Similar osmotic effects to those associated with galactosaemia occur and lead to cataract formation [13]. There

are no systemic manifestations of the disease and patients usually enjoy normal general health. If the deficiency is recognized early enough, however, the cataracts are reversible by the use of a galactose-free diet.

3.4.4 Lowe's syndrome

This disease is due to an X-linked recessive characteristic with an unknown enzyme defect and is possibly due to deficient amino acid transport [14]. The syndrome is associated with bilateral nuclear cataracts [15], microphakia and severe congenital glaucoma [9]. The latter is due to malformation of the anterior chamber angle or to subluxated lenses. Other ocular abnormalities include iris malformation and a blue sclera, which is a manifestation of scleral thinning. There is a poor prognosis for full visual recovery after cataract surgery. Systemic manifestations of the disease include mental and growth retardation with hypotonia, vitamin-D-associated rickets and metabolic acidosis.

3.4.5 Myotonic dystrophy

The disorder is inherited as an autosomal dominant trait. Early cataracts are characteristic and consist of multicoloured refractile bodies scattered among finer dust-like opacities in the cortex and subcapsular area. A granular posterior subcapsular cataract develops later in the disease [16], with the nucleus remaining clear. Other ocular abnormalities may include optic atrophy and retinal degeneration [12]. Associated systemic findings include dystrophic changes in muscles, along with impaired contraction and relaxation.

3.4.6 Hypoglycaemia

Neonatal hypoglycaemia occurs in approximately 20% of newborn infants, the incidence being significantly higher in premature infants [12]. Blood sugar levels of 20 mg dl^{-1} or less, may cause repeated episodes of drowsiness, unconsciousness and convulsions. Repeated hypoglycaemic episodes may lead to the appearance of a characteristic lamellar cataract in the 2–3-year-old child [12]. Treatment of this condition is aimed at the restoration and maintenance of normal blood glucose levels.

3.5 Adult cataract

Four main types of age-related cataract morphology are recognized:

(a) cortical cataracts, appearing as spokes or base-out wedges of opacity in the anterior and/or posterior cortex (Section 3.5.1);
(b) anterior subcapsular cataracts, appearing as plaque-like opacities at the anterior pole (Section 3.5.2);
(c) posterior subcapsular cataracts, appearing as granular plaque-like opacities at the posterior pole (Section 3.5.2);
(d) nuclear cataracts, characterized by a homogeneous yellow or brunescent coloration and light scatter (Section 3.5.3).

Fluctuation in the refractive index of a cataractous lens creates foci of light scattering and a loss of transparency. In cortical and subcapsular cataracts, light scattering is believed to occur as a result of the interfibrillar accumulation of protein-deficient lakes of fluid [17]. Wide discrepancies in the index of refraction of the interfibrillar spaces and the fibre cytoplasm lead to light scattering at the interface. Light scattering also occurs from large protein aggregates linked to the cell membrane by disulphide bonds. In nuclear cataract, light is scattered by large soluble protein aggregates with molecular weights in excess of $5 \times 106\,\mathrm{Da}$ [12]. The mechanisms responsible for these cataractous changes are discussed below.

3.5.1 Cortical(cuneiform) cataract

The wedge shaped opacity is located in the cortex of the lens, usually affecting the anterior cortex more than the posterior [4]. Since the base of the wedge or spoke is located in the periphery of the lens, vision is not affected until the apices of the wedges are sufficiently dense within the pupillary area or cross the visual axis.

Wedges are generally first seen in the inferior or inferionasal aspect of the cortex. The progression of cortical opacities varies. Much of this variation seems to depend on the degree of hydration of the lens. If the lens becomes hydrated, the opacities may progress rapidly, with the lens showing signs of intumescence caused by the presence of many fluid vacuoles and clefts between lens fibres. The fluid, derived from the aqueous, can separate the fibres in either a radial or lamellar manner. In radial separation, fluid follows the natural course of the lens fibres, resulting in wedge-shaped clefts. As the water clefts opacify, the typical picture of cortical spokes emerges. Lamellar separation appears as numerous fine parallel lines, often running in a near-horizontal direction in a quadrant of the lens [9]. At this stage of maturity, the anterior cortex of the lens appears bright silver–white to dark-grey or yellow. It is not possible to observe the posterior portion of the lens in this state, although other cataract forms may coexist [9]. In other cases, the opaque spokes may be small, discrete and somewhat evenly distributed around the lens periphery. Alternatively, several spokes may coalesce in one section of the lens.

When the cataractous changes occur without hydration of the lens, they may progress very slowly. The spokes eventually invade the pupillary area, however, usually causing the anterior cortex to become totally opaque. At this stage the lens is referred to as a mature cataract.

Deep cortical cataracts are sometimes classified separately as supranuclear opacities.

3.5.2 Subcapsular cataract

This cataract is also referred to as cupuliform, describing the classic concave disc-shaped appearance of the opacity in its mature form, when viewed stereoscopically. Granular opacities in the subcapsular clear zone occur in some forms of age-related cataract and in cataract secondary to eye disease, radiation and trauma [17].

The cataracts are usually located centrally within the pupillary area and in the posterior cortex immediately adjacent to the capsule. The combination of its location and optical density causes a marked effect on VA. Anterior subcapsular cataracts are less common.

Subcapsular cataracts are frequently caused by damage to the subcapsular epithelium. The resultant histological changes are similar, whatever the cause of the injury and are due to the proliferation of epithelial cells.

In the development of a posterior subcapsular cataract, the first change that occurs is the posterior migration of epithelial cells [18]. Vacuoles are frequently interspersed amongst the opacities. It has been suggested that mechanisms other than posterior migration of equatorial cells may account for some kinds of posterior subcapsular cataracts [19]. For example, osmotic imbalance could be responsible for the opacities.

Subcapsular cataracts tend to progress during a period of months if the initial insult was severe, or if the cause is not removed. Cortical or nuclear sclerotic cataract may coexist with subcapsular cataract [4].

3.5.3 Nuclear sclerotic cataract

The nucleus tends to remain free of opacity until the onset of age-related nuclear sclerotic cataract. As the refractive index increases and the lens becomes more sclerotic with age, the nucleus changes from appearing optically empty to becoming optically visible. The transition from a normal ageing nucleus to nuclear sclerosis is not sharply defined. This process usually begins between the ages of 50 and 60, with increased incidence in patients in their 60s and 70s [4].

Clinically, the nuclear sclerotic cataract is encountered (either alone or in combination with other age-related lens changes) more frequently than any other age-related cataract [4]. It has been described as the most common form of age-related cataract to cause reduced central VA [4]. Nuclear sclerosis may also be secondary to trauma or uveitis [9].

3.6 Cataract and diabetes mellitus (DM)

An association between cataract and DM in the human population has been suspected for about two centuries. This has resulted in considerable laboratory research into the development of animal models, in which the eye disease process could be studied in detail. From these studies, it was observed that DM, produced by either pancreatomy or chemical destruction of β-cells of the pancreas, led to cataracts in dogs, rats and monkeys. The rapidity of cataract development reflected the severity of the DM. The diabetic complications, therefore, appeared to be directly related to the blood glucose level.

Numerous studies have been made on the relationship between cataract and DM. Some results suggest that DM is a significant cataractogenic stress which, in combination with other age-related stresses, may lead to earlier maturation of cataract. Cotlier *et al.* [20] found that there is excellent correlation of cataract progression with age in both diabetic and non-diabetic cataracts. Progression in diabetics was the more rapid of the two. Schwab *et al.* [21] reported the overall rate (adjusted for age and sex) of cataract surgery, in a population of Pima Indians, to be 2.2 times higher in diabetics than in non-diabetics. The rate of cataract surgery in insulin-treated diabetics was found to be approximately 5 times that of non-diabetics. The rate of cataract surgery increased with increasing duration of DM. Prevalence studies have shown an association of lens opacities and cataract with DM [22]. The extent to which relatively minor lens opacities are early evidence of visually significant age-related cataract is unknown.

Other workers have suggested that the apparent excess of diabetics undergoing cataract surgery may, in fact, be due to early detection and referral of patients already under medical surveillance. A study by Skalka and Prchal [23] failed to demonstrate a significant association between the presence of DM and lens opacities. DM, however, appeared to be associated with increased risk of visually significant lens opacities. Race, degree of metabolic control and age of onset of DM were not found to be correlated with cataract formation.

There is, therefore, a great degree of controversy in the literature, with results often appearing contradictory and confusing. On occasions, conclusions have been drawn from uncontrolled or biased studies, where standardizing methods of examination and selection of controls have been ignored. Nevertheless, the existence of true diabetic cataract and a high proportion of diabetics with age-related cataract, cannot be ignored.

3.7 Diabetic cataract

The true diabetic cataract is a rare complication of DM in the young. It usually occurs rapidly, often with sudden myopia, occurring bilaterally in the superficial layers of the lens cortex. It is potentially reversible during the early stages [12].

3.8 Age-related cataract in DM

Age-related cataract in older diabetics is far more common. In the Oxford region, Caird [24] found that diabetics were 5 times more likely to undergo cataract surgery than non diabetics. In a more recent survey, it was found that 44% of cataract patients had an abnormal glucose tolerance curve [25]. In a large study of 1300 diabetics [26], cataract was found to be the second most frequent cause of visual loss after maculopathy. Caird *et al.* [27] observed that in the 7% of new cases of DM, which were observed by ophthalmologists, more than 50% were diagnosed as a result of visual symptoms due to cataract.

Three major mechanisms have been proposed to explain the formation of sugar cataract:

(a) the polyol theory (Section 3.8.1);
(b) auto-oxidation of sugars (Section 3.8.2);
(c) non-enzymatic protein glycosylation (Section 3.8.3).

3.8.1 The polyol theory

The polyol (or sugar alcohol) theory is derived from the observation that lenses of hyper-glycaemic animals developed areas of increased light scattering or opacification [28]. When examined biochemically, these lenses were found to contain greater than normal levels of sorbitol, the sugar alcohol formed by the reduction of the aldehyde group of glucose by AR. The enzymes AR and sorbitol dehydrogenase constitute the sorbitol pathway in tissues containing these enzymes.

In cells that permit glucose entry without the action of insulin, intracellular glucose levels follow the extracellular levels. In periods of hyperglycaemia, high intracellular glucose levels result in increased AR activity and accumulation of sorbitol. Sorbitol dehydrogenase cannot keep pace with the rising levels of its substrate. Since sorbitol does not readily pass through cell membranes, its accumulation within cells creates a net inward movement of water in an attempt to restore osmotic equilibrium [29]. Instead of normalizing the situation, however, osmotic swelling of the cells results in an alteration of membrane integrity and transport activity. This in turn, leads to the loss of amino acids, inositol and K^+ ions and an influx of Na^+ ions. Further lens fibre cell swelling results in loss of cell membrane continuity and loss of critical metabolites and proteins. Ultimately, the cells die and liquefy, leaving vacuoles in their place [30].

In summary, accumulation of sorbitol formed via the AR reaction produces an osmotic imbalance between the lens and aqueous humour. This causes an influx of water, followed by swelling, disruption of membranes, leakage of amino acids and hydration.

The osmotic hypothesis, based on early evidence from animal studies, has been subjected to several criticisms when applied to human diabetic cataract formation [17]. The osmotic effect of accumulated polyol can possibly play a role in the formation of cataract in the galactose-fed rat but may be of minor importance in the human diabetic patient. Osmotically significant levels of sorbitol have never been found in the human lens, which contains only barely detectable levels of AR. The human lens has a relatively high polyol dehydrogenase content. Any sorbitol formed would, therefore, be rapidly converted into fructose to be further metabolized [31].

3.8.2 Auto-oxidation of sugars

A second possible mechanism of sugar cataract formation is that of spontaneous oxidation of sugars. The by-products of these oxidations then react non-enzymatically with the lens proteins [17]. No proof of this mechanism *in vivo* has, as yet, been published in the literature.

Auto-oxidation does not occur in glucose or ribose but could possibly occur in some of the rarer sugars present. Glyceraldehyde, for example, has been shown to breakdown spontaneously in air [32] and may therefore possibly breakdown *in vivo*. Auto-oxidation products of glyceraldehyde include highly reactive free radicals such as peroxide and superoxide (see Section 2.7.1.2). No specific damage by free radicals to lens conformation and structure has been demonstrated, however.

In conclusion, the role of auto-oxidation in cataract formation is uncertain [17]. Free radical production from glucose and ribose is not detectable. The reactions of glucose and its major metabolites are expected to be more relevant than glyceraldehyde to the aetiology of cataract in diabetics.

3.8.3 Non-enzymatic glycosylation

The third possible mechanism of cataractogenesis also involves non-enzymatic reactions with the lens proteins. The extent of non-enzymatic glycosylation in the lens has been shown to increase in DM [33]. Stevens *et al.* [34] reported that the reaction of glucose and glucose 6-phosphate with lens proteins induced an opalescence that was partly dependent on disulphide cross-linking. It was suggested that non-enzymatic glycosylation altered the conformation of the proteins, promoting disulphide cross-linking and therefore protein aggregation. The change in conformation has been confirmed and measured by circular dichroism [35].

In conclusion, non-enzymatic glycosylation and the polyol theory both seem to be important pathways in the aetiology of cataract in diabetics. The sugar auto-oxidation theory has not yet been satisfactorily established. Discussion of all three mechanisms continues 30 years or so after the polyol theory was first proposed.

3.9 Hypocalcaemic (tetanic) cataract

These cataracts occur in association with infantile tetany or with hypoparathyroidism or rickets in other age groups. It is believed that calcium is necessary for the maintenance of membrane integrity and that calcium deficiency leads to membrane disruption and increased permeability [12]. (See also Section 2.7.4). In the adult, acquired or surgical hypoparathyroidism is associated with the formation of highly refractile punctate opacities initially in the subcapsular area. After treatment, the punctate opacities sink into the nucleus, where they may form a lamellar cataract [9]. Other ocular manifestations of the condition may include papilloedema, diplopia, photophobia and strabismus [12].

3.10 Cataract secondary to other systemic and ophthalmological cataractogenic stresses

The discussion is limited to those factors that are encountered with some frequency in clinical practice.

3.10.1 Corticosteroids

Either long-term or high-dose short-term oral administration of corticosteroids may be followed by the development of a posterior subcapsular opacity, after a latent period of 1–2 years. Topical administration of steroids can also cause subcapsular cataract [9]. The opacity generally remains as a lamellar cataract [9] if the steroids are withdrawn.

3.10.2 Radiation cataract

Ionizing forms of radiation (including X-rays, γ-rays, β-rays and neutrons) have been found to be cataractogenic [9,12]. Exposure to X-rays during the first trimester of pregnancy can cause congenital cataracts [9]. Ionizing radiation affects the germinal epithelium at the lens equator [36,37]. The opacity is therefore more pronounced in younger lenses which have a high mitotic rate. The damaged epithelium gives rise to a granular material that moves centripetally in the subcapsular region towards the lens poles, especially the posterior pole [38]. This granular material is recognized after a latent period of several months or years.

Other non-ionizing forms of electromagnetic energy can also cause cataract. Chronic exposure to infra-red radiation, such as occurs in glassblowers and furnace workers, may give rise to posterior subcapsular cataract. The cataract is probably caused by exposure of the iris pigment epithelium and consequently the lens epithelium, to extreme heat. This frequently results in a thickened lens capsule and exfoliation. Ultraviolet (UV) and microwave radiation have also been implicated in cataract formation [39]. Laser radiation has been found to cause a localized capsular opacity in human lenses [40].

Repetitive exposure of the human lens to the near-UV light (300–400 nm) of sunlight, may be a possible cause of lens opacification [41,42]. This results from the absorption of radiant energy by yellow chromophores, present in both free form [43] and lens proteins [44].

3.10.3 Traumatic cataract

Both penetrating and non-penetrating physical injuries can cause a variety of traumatic lens changes ranging from discrete punctate opacities to total lens involvement [45].

Concussion of the lens, without rupture of the capsule, may result in a cataract that is initially subcapsular [46] and commonly has a star-shaped appearance. This stellate (rose-shaped) opacity is the most typical clinical lens change occurring as a result of injury [4]. Complete opacification of the lens with a uniform milky appearance may occur as a result of concussion but is usually associated with perforation of the lens capsule [4]. A small capsular tear may seal itself, resulting in only a localized opacity of capsule and cortex [9].

Traumatic cataract has been reported to occur as either an early or late response to trauma.

In the early type of cataract, the opacity may develop hours, weeks or months after the injury. The characteristic feathery appearance of the opacity results from the formation of small fluid droplets between the radiating lens fibres. The effect of these petals on vision is determined by the density of the opacities. The opacity progresses towards the deep cortex, or infantile nucleus, as the lens grows. In a few cases of severe trauma, when growth is inhibited, the opacity remains subcapsular [9].

The late-onset stellate opacity occurs years after the trauma. It is found deep within the cortex or adult nucleus, with an overlying zone of clear cortex.

Other energy sources such as electricity [47] have also been found to cause traumatic cataract.

3.10.4 Cataract secondary to local eye disease (complicated cataract)

This term applies to the development of cataracts secondary to local inflammatory, degenerative and anoxic conditions. The most common cause of this cataract type is iridocyclitis, usually associated with posterior synechiae [9]. Such cataracts are also manifestations of chronic uveitis, including Fuchs' heterochromic cyclitis and Still's disease. Degenerative conditions include long-standing retinal detachment, retinitis pigmentosa and chronic glaucoma [9]. These cataracts may also result from intraocular tumours, ocular ischaemia and may occur after local surgery, especially glaucoma filtering procedures and retinal detachment surgery.

Complicated cataracts are characteristically located in a posterior subcapsular site but may take the form of nuclear sclerosis or cupuliform cataract, both of which are indistinguishable from their age-related or traumatic forms. The subcapsular cataract consists of granules and vacuoles that often appear to extend into the cortex, anterior to the main opacity. The most anteriorly placed opacities were the first to be laid down, at which time they were themselves subcapsular [9]. The total depth of the opacity is, therefore, related to the length of time it has been present. The condition eventually progresses to mature cataract unless the causative disease process is treated.

3.10.5 Miscellaneous secondary cataract types

3.10.5.1 Down's syndrome

Cataracts occur as an ocular manifestation of Down's syndrome in about 75% of patients [10]. Congenital cataracts are present in the foetal nucleus in a small percentage of Down's patients [10]. It is more usual for scattered punctate and flake-like opacities to develop in the cortex early in life [48], lens sutures frequently appearing more prominent and grey.

3.10.5.2 Dermatogenic cataract

The most common cutaneous disease associated with cataract is atopic dermatitis [9], an allergic disorder with a familial tendency. Bilateral subcapsular cataract, generally posterior, develops in approximately 10% of patients in their 20s [9].

References

1. Merin, S. Congenital cataracts. In *Genetic and Metabolic Eye Disease* (edited by M.F. Goldberg), Little, Brown and Company, Boston (1974)
2. Fraser, G.R. and Friedman, A.I. *The Causes of Blindness in Childhood*, Johns Hopkins Press, Baltimore (1967)
3. Chylack, L.T. and Cheng, H.M. Clinical implications of research on lens and cataract. In *The Ocular Lens* (edited by H. Maisel), Marcel Dekker, Inc., New York, pp. 439–466 (1985)
4. Amos, J.F. and Norden, L.C. The eye not correctable to 20/20. In *Diagnosis and Management in Vision Care* (edited by J.F. Amos), Butterworths, Boston, pp. 263–312 (1987)
5. Parks, M.M. Posterior lens capsulectomy during primary cataract surgery in children. *Ophthalmology*, **90**, 344–345 (1983)
6. Rogers, G.L., Tishler, C.L. and Tsou, B.H. Visual acuities in infants with congenital cataracts operated on prior to 6 months of age. *Archives of Ophthalmology*, **99**, 999–1003 (1981)
7. Gelbart, S.S., Hoyt, C.S., Jastrebski, G. *et al.* Long-term visual results in bilateral congenital cataracts.

American Journal of Ophthalmology, **93,** 615–621 (1982)

8. Merin, S. and Crawford, J.S. The aetiology of congenital cataracts: A survey of 386 cases. *Canadian Journal of Ophthalmology,* **6,** 178–182 (1971)

9. Berger, B.B., Emery, J.M., Brown, N.V. The lens, cataract and its management. In *Principles and Practice of Ophthalmology* (edited by G.A Peyman, D.R. Sanders and M.F. Goldberg), W.B. Saunders Company, Philadelphia, pp. 489–632 (1980)

10. Alden, E.R., Kalina, R.E. and Hodson, W.B. Transient cataracts in low birth weight infants. *Journal of Paediatrics and Child Health,* **82,** 314–318 (1973)

11. Gregg, N.M. Congenital cataract following German measles in the mother. *Transactions of the Ophthalmological Societies of Australia,* **3,** 35–42 (1941)

12. Chylack, L.T. The crystalline lens and cataract. In *Manual of Ocular Diagnosis and Therapy* (edited by D. Pavan-Langston), Little, Brown and Company, Boston and Toronto, pp. 117–138 (1985)

13. Isselbacher, K.J. In *The Metabolic Basis of Inherited Disease* (edited by J.B. Stanbury, J.B. Wyngaarden and D.S. Frederichson), McGraw-Hill, New York, pp. 174–195 (1972)

14. Boger, W.P. and Petersen, R.A. Paediatric ophthalmology. In *Manual of Ocular Diagnosis and Therapy* (edited by D. Pavan-Langston), Little, Brown and Company, Boston and Toronto, pp. 231–274 (1985)

15. Curtin, V.T., Joyce, E.E. and Ballin, W. *American Journal of Ophthalmology,* **64,** 533–543 (1967)

16. Pescia, G. and Emery, A.E.H. *Journal de Genetique Humaine,* **24,** 227–234 (1976)

17. Harding, J. *Cataract: Biochemistry, Epidemiology and Pharmacology,* Chapman and Hall, London (1991)

18. Streeten, B.W. and Eshaghian, J. Human posterior subcapsular cataract. A gross and flat preparation study. *Archives of Ophthalmology,* **96,** 1653–1658 (1978)

19. Harding, C.V., Susan, S.R. and Lo, W.K. The structure of the human cataractous lens. In *The Ocular Lens* (edited by H. Maisel), Marcel Dekker, Inc., New York, pp. 367–404 (1985)

20. Cotlier, E., Fagadau, W. and Cicchetti, D.V. Methods for evaluation of medical therapy of age-related and diabetic cataracts. *Transactions of the Ophthalmological Societies of the United Kingdom,* **102,** 416–422 (1982)

21. Schwab, I.R., Davison, C.R. and Hoshiwara, I. Incidence of cataract extraction in Pima Indians. Diabetes as a risk factor. *Archives of Ophthalmology,* **103,** 208–212 (1985)

22. Nielsen, N.V. and Vinding, T. The prevalence of cataract in insulin-dependent and non-insulin-dependent diabetes mellitus. *Acta Ophthalmologica,* **62,** 595–602 (1984)

23. Skalka, H.W. and Prchal, J.T. The effect of diabetes mellitus and diabetic therapy on cataract formation. *Ophthalmology,* **88,** 117–124 (1981)

24. Caird, F.I. In *The Human Lens in Relation to Cataract* (edited by K. Elliot and D.W. Fitzsimmons) (Ciba Symposium 19), Elsevier, London, pp. 281–301 (1973)

25. Crabbe, M.J.C. and Harding, J.J. Diabetic and galactosemic cataracts. *Transactions of the Ophthalmological Societies of the United Kingdom,* **102,** 342–345 (1982)

26. Mitchell, P. The prevalence of diabetic retinopathy: The study of 1300 diabetics from Newcastle and the Hunter Valley. *Australian Journal of Ophthalmology,* **8,** 341–346 (1980)

27. Caird, F.I., Burditt, A.F. and Draper, G.J. Diabetic retinopathy. *Diabetics,* **17** (3), 121–123 (1968)

28. Van Heyningen, R. Formation of polyols by the lens of the rat with 'sugar' cataract. *Nature,* **184,** 194–195 (1959)

29. Kinoshita, J.H., Merola, L.O. and Dikmak, E. Osmotic changes in experimental galactose cataracts. *Experimental Eye Research,* **1,** 405–410 (1962)

30. Varma S. In *Current Topics in Eye Research,* Academic Press, New York, vol. 3, pp. 91–155 (1980)

31. Jedziniak, J.A., Chylack, L.T. and Cheng, H.M. The sorbitol pathway in the human lens: aldose reductase and polyol dehydrogenase. *Investigative Ophthalmology and Visual Science,* **20,** 314–326 (1981)

32. Wolff, S.P., Crabbe, M.J.C. and Thornalley, P.J. The autoxidation of glyceraldehyde and other simple monosaccharides. *Experientia,* **40,** 244–246 (1984)

33. Harding, J.J. Nonenzymic covalent post-translational modification of proteins *in vivo*. *Advances in Protein Chemistry,* **37,** 247–334 (1985)

34. Stevens, V.J., Rouzer, C.A., Monnier, V.M. and Cerami, A. Diabetic cataract formation: potential role of glycosylation of lens crystallins. *Proceedings of the National Academy of Sciences of the United States of America,* **75,** 2918–2922 (1978)

35. Liang, J.N. and Rossi, M.T. *In vitro* non-enzymatic glycation and formation of browning products in the bovine lens alpha-crystallin. *Experimental Eye Research,* **50,** 367–371 (1990)

36. Kimura, S. and Ikui, H. Atom-bomb radiation cataract. *American Journal of Ophthalmology,* **34,** 811–818 (1951)

37. Cogan, D. and Donaldson, D. Clinical and pathological characteristics of radiation cataract. *Archives of Ophthalmology,* **47,** 55–63 (1952)

38. Rafferty, N.S., Goossens, B.A. and March, W.F. Ultrastructure of human traumatic cataracts. *American Journal of Ophthalmology,* **78,** 985–995 (1974)

39. Zaret, M.M. and Snyder, W.Z. Cataracts and avionic radiations. *British Journal of Ophthalmology,* **61,** 380–384 (1977)

40. Pollack, I.P. and Patz, A. Argon laser iridotomy: An experimental and clinical study. *Ophthalmic Surgery,* **7,** 22–30 (1976)

41. Zigman, S., Datiles, M. and Torczynski, E. Sunlight and human cataracts. *Investigative Ophthalmology and Visual Science,* **18,** 462–467 (1979)

42. Zigman, S., Schultz, J. and Yulo, T. Possible roles of near UV light in the cataractous process. *Experimental Eye Research,* **15,** 201–208 (1973)

43. Van Heyningen, R. Fluorescent compounds of the human lens. In *The Human Lens in relation to Cataract* (Ciba Symposium, **19**), Elsevier, London pp. 151–171 (1973)

44. Dillon, J.P. and Spector, A. Aerobic and anaerobic photochemical modification of lens protein analyzed by synchronous scan fluorescent techniques. *Investigative Ophthalmology and Visual Science (Supplement)*, 127 (1979)

45. Duke-Elder, S. and MacFaul, P.A. Injuries. I. Mechanical injuries. In *System of Ophthalmology* (edited by S. Duke-Elder), CV Mosby Co., St Louis, vol. 14, pp. 130–142 (1972)

46. Davidson, M. Lens lesions in contusion: A medicolegal study. *American Journal of Ophthalmology*, **23**, 252–258 (1940)

47. Fraunfelder, F. and Hanna, C. Electric cataracts: Part II. *Archives of Ophthalmology*, **87**, 184–191 (1972)

48. Ginsberg, J., Bofinger, M. and Roush, J.A.R. Pathologic features of the eye in Down's syndrome with relationship to other chromosomal anomalies. *American Journal of Ophthalmology*, **83**, 874–880 (1977)

4

Signs, symptoms and patient management

Janet Hesler

4.1 General signs and symptoms

Those of us who are fortunate enough not to be affected by cataract can but guess what it is like. Patients with cataract can describe their vision but they cannot be relied upon to give a good descriptive account. This depends on their recollection of the visual quality prior to the onset of cataract and this is likely to be particularly unreliable because the progression of cataract is usually slow.

A patient with cataract can describe a variety of symptoms, the most common of which is a slowly progressive painless deterioration in visual acuity (VA). This is frequently described as a film or fog which has 'grown over the eyes' or as having the sensation of a grease mark which cannot be removed from a spectacle lens. The vision often varies with the lighting. Depending upon the size and location of the lens opacity, vision may be better under dim rather than bright illumination or vice versa. The patient may report that she or he can read near print without the previously required reading spectacles, often recounted as 'second sight'. The problem of monocular diplopia could be an additional symptom. Halos and stars are commonly seen around lights as a result of diffraction. These are usually white/yellow in colour and thus can be differentiated from the more typical rainbow coloured phenomenon described in acute glaucoma.

The most significant basic effect of cataract on vision is that of light scattering. Light scattered within the eye by cataract acts as a veiling luminance which reduces the contrast of the image received by the retina and thus makes the object of regard more difficult to perceive. As the cataract progresses, the amount of light scatter also progresses, giving rise to the typical symptom of painless gradual deterioration in vision.

It is sometimes possible to obtain a clear view of the retina using a direct ophthalmoscope and a dilated pupil, even though the eye has poor VA. Miller [1] has fully described this phenomenon.

A more detailed account of signs and symptoms is given later in this chapter.

4.2 Examination

The fact that several of the symptoms reported by cataract patients can be due to conditions other than cataract requires the patient to undergo a thorough ocular examination. A reduction in acuity due to retinal or neural disease can be detected by certain subjective tests, for example, displacement threshold hyperacuities and laser interferometry (see Chapter 6). The location and density of any lens opacity, the probable cause and the likelihood of progression, can be determined by examination using an ophthalmoscope and slit-lamp biomicroscope with a widely dilated pupil. Also, the optical significance of the opacity can be objectively evaluated by this technique. The clinician must have a good knowledge of the human crystalline lens and its various landmarks, in order to carry out a good examination.

The lens capsule can often be seen during slit lamp examination. If the pupil is widely dilated, a view of the zonular fibres can also be obtained. These have the appearance of hundreds of taut cobwebs extending towards the equatorial region of the lens. Unless the lens is particularly cataractous, the nucleus, the anterior and posterior Y sutures and the posterior capsule of the lens can usually be distinguished quite easily using a slit optical section. In addition, if the pupil is widely dilated, the anterior portion of the vitreous humour can be seen. As the eye moves, the vitreous appears to 'shimmer', thus distinguishing it from the crystalline lens material.

The optical section technique is particularly useful for the assessment of nuclear changes and for deciding on the position of lens opacities. However, the retroillumination technique is a superior approach when viewing cortical and posterior subcapsular (PSC) changes. The retro-illumination technique can be performed by using an ophthalmoscope with a plano lens in its observation system and viewing an eye with a dilated pupil from a distance of about 60 cm. However, better magnification can be obtained by viewing the lens with a slit lamp.

The location of an opacity within the lens determines its classification. Those in the nucleus are nuclear cataracts. Similarly, those in the cortex are cortical and so on. The morphological types of age-related cataract fall largely into three basic categories: cortical spoke (sometimes also called cuneiform), nuclear and PSC (see Chapter 3). Cataracts have been classified into these three categories for the purpose of clinical studies [2]. These cataract types can be graded clinically [2,3] and can be measured photographically [4–6]. The differential diagnosis of cataract is given elsewhere but, briefly, cortical cataract appears as base-out wedge shapes with the apex pointing towards the centre of the pupil (Figure 4.1).

Nuclear cataract causes both brunescence (Figure 4.2a) and white scattering (Figure 4.2b). Brunescence is best seen by viewing the reflected brown/yellow light from the posterior capsule when viewed in optical section.

PSC cataract is usually positioned in the central pupillary region on, or close to, the visual axis and has a granular/plaque appearance arranged in a saucer shaped pattern (Figure 4.3).

4.3 Specific signs and symptoms

Our current understanding of the characteristics of cataract enable us to illustrate the types of visual disability that a cataract patient may experience. In this section, the visual disability caused by cataract is simulated by the use of a 'cataractous camera'. This is a standard SLR camera which has been equipped with coloured and neutral density filters to represent various cataract types. These filters are used in front of the camera lens to produce photographs which give a fair portrayal of the visual disability.

There are nine demonstrable ways in which vision is affected by cataract. These are:

(1) myopic shift;
(2) monocular diplopia;
(3) astigmatism;
(4) contrast sensitivity reduction;
(5) glare;
(6) colour shift;
(7) reduced light transmission;
(8) field loss;
(9) VA reduction

4.3.1 Myopic shift

The normal ageing process of the human crystalline lens causes the eye to become progressively more hypermetropic [7]. Normal ageing patients and those developing cortical or PSC cataract without nuclear change show this continued hypermetropic shift. However, during nuclear cataract progression, the lens nucleus becomes more compacted and hardened. This causes the refractive index of the nucleus to increase, thus rendering the eye more myopic. It is possible to predict that an ageing person is developing nuclear cataract if they show a 0.50 D myopic shift between refractions 2 years apart [8]. The myopia caused by the development of nuclear cataract, therefore, can more than offset the normal ageing hypermetropic shift. Such hypermetropic patients are usually initially delighted at the change in their ametropia, since they are able to see with weaker lenses. As the nuclear sclerosis progresses, other more adverse effects of the cataract, such as light scatter, cause degradation of the retinal image.

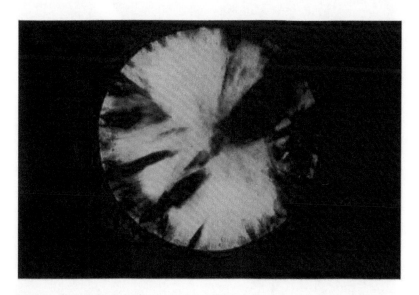

Figure 4.1 Cortical spoke cataract (courtesy of N.A.P. Brown and the Optician).

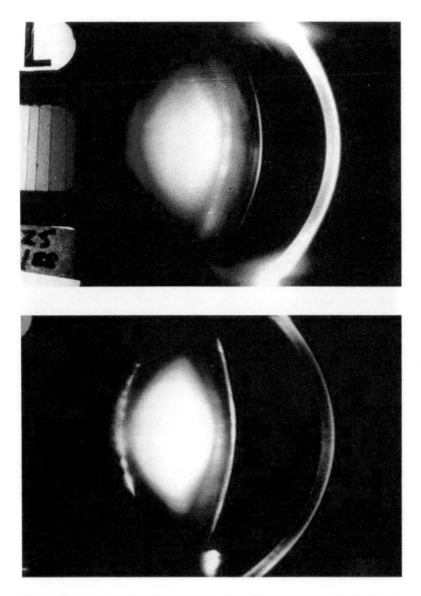

Figure 4.2(a) Nuclear brunescence (courtesy of N.A.P. Brown and the Optician); (b) nuclear white scatter (courtesy of N.A.P. Brown and the Optician).

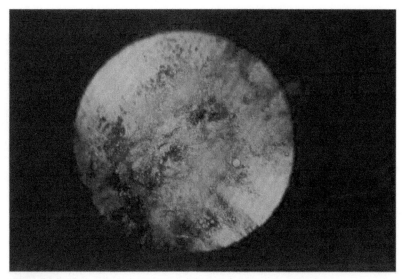

Figure 4.3 Posterior subcapsular cataract (courtesy of N.A.P. Brown).

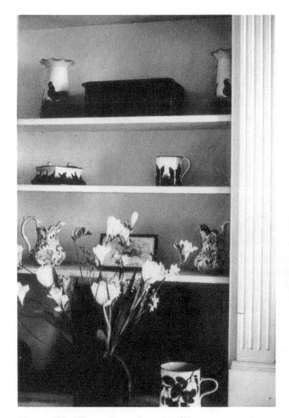 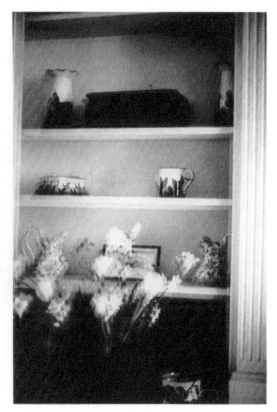

Figure 4.4(a) Normal eye view of a living room shelf (courtesy of N.A.P. Brown); (b) Monocular diplopia caused by 1 Δ of displacement (courtesy of N.A.P. Brown).

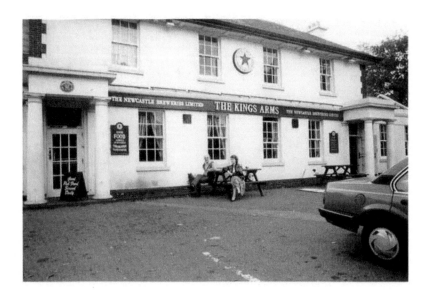

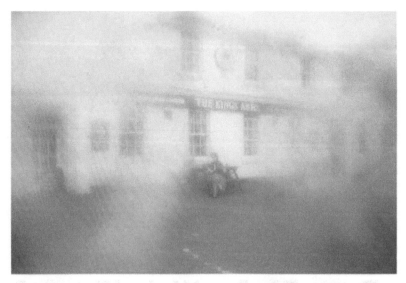

Figure 4.5(a) A public house viewed with a normal lens; (b) The same scene with cortical cataract. The high-contrast detail of the pub sign remains well seen, but the low-contrast features, such as the person on the left, are not easily detected.

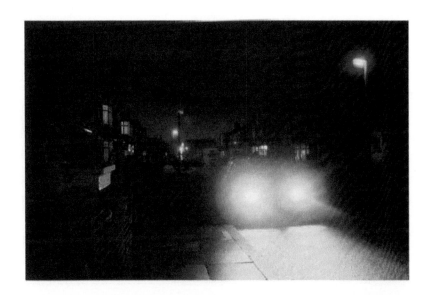

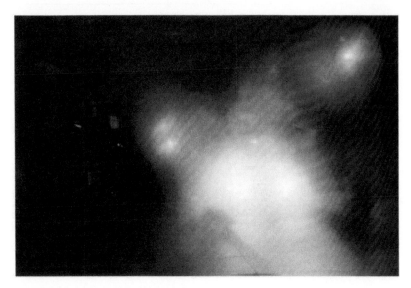

Figure 4.6(a) A street scene at night viewed by a normal eye; (b) The same street scene viewed with a cortical cataract.

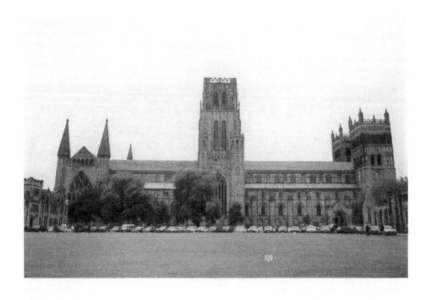

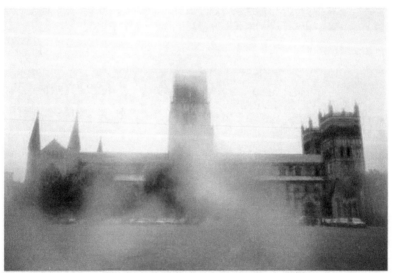

Figure 4.7(a) A view of Durham Cathedral with a normal eye. (b) The same view seen through a cortical spoke cataract.

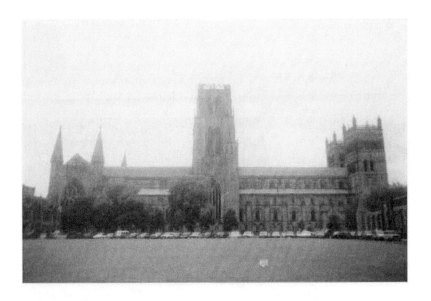

Figure 4.7(c) Durham Cathedral seen with a lens having nuclear brunescence only. (d) The more usual situation in which brunescence coexists with nuclear scatter.

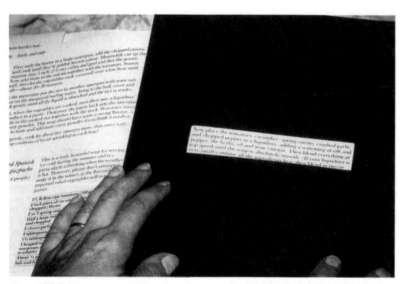

Figure 4.8 A typoscope: used to reduce the amount of light reflected from the page.

4.3.2 Monocular diplopia

Any small defect in the optical system of the human eye can cause great visual disturbance. In cataract, where the refractive index of the crystalline lens changes unevenly, it is easy to understand why monocular diplopia occurs. A localized area of differing refractive index may act like a prism and divide the light rays to produce two images. Monocular diplopia is particularly common in the presence of cortical spokes or waterclefts, although it can occur in nuclear cataract where the nucleus and cortex produce separate images.

Only a small prismatic effect is required to cause the double image. Figure 4.4(a) is a normal view of a living room shelf. Figure 4.4(b) is the same scene taken with a prism of only 1 prism dioptre (Δ) covering part of the camera lens. The amount of diplopia caused by this small prism is very noticeable.

A pinhole can be used to ascertain the cause of the monocular diplopia. That caused by refractive change, as in cataract, will be eliminated with the pinhole in place. Monocular diplopia with a retinal aetiology will remain when the pinhole is used.

It is very difficult to eliminate monocular diplopia with spectacle lenses. Nevertheless, the patient may be less aware of the doubled image when wearing the best possible optical correction.

4.3.3 Astigmatism

Although there has been little formal research into this aspect of vision through cataracts, clinical experience tells us that astigmatic shifts do occur during cataract progression. As already discussed, in cataract, the refractive index of the lens changes at an uneven rate and it is this that is likely to cause the astigmatic fluctuations. In particular, experienced refractionists feel that cortical spoke cataracts cause the most astigmatic change.

Objective methods of determining the astigmatic correction, such as the retinoscope and the auto refractor, are usually unhelpful with cataract patients. Subjective methods of refraction prove to be more useful in determining the cylinder power and axis. Since patients will often be helped by quite small changes in their astigmatic correction, it is well worth taking some time to search for new astigmatic errors.

4.3.4 Contrast sensitivity

Contrast sensitivity (CS) is a familiar tool in vision research and is now becoming accepted as a necessary part of the clinical assessment of visual function. CS is recognized as providing a more comprehensive record of a patient's visual performance than VA. While VA measures the threshold of resolution of small high-contrast targets, CS measures the visibility of both large and small targets at various contrast levels. The reason why CS provides a more thorough evaluation of visual performance is better understood by using hearing as an analogy. The quality of sound is not determined purely by the highest frequency that can be heard, just as the quality of vision is not determined by the smallest letters that can be resolved. Visual performance can, therefore, be better assessed by measuring the thresholds to contrast through a range of target sizes (spatial frequencies).

The predominant cause of visual loss in the cataractous eye is light scatter. This produces a veiling luminance that is superimposed on the retinal image, causing a contrast lowering effect of the object of regard. Theoretically, therefore, it would seem likely that CS measurement would lend itself readily to the assessment of visual function. In practice, this has been shown to be the case, with several investigators finding that CS measurement is more useful than VA measurement in cataract patients [9–11], and that CS measurements relate directly to the visual impairment experienced by cataract patients [12,13]. The conventional Snellen VA chart is, in effect, a very high contrast high spatial frequency test which corresponds to few items in the real world. As such, CS testing is more informative than VA with regard to the cataract patient's overall visual performance. All cataracts lower CS, and the PSC cataract has been shown to induce the greatest loss [14]. The performance of the eye with cataract is reduced throughout the spatial frequency range. When the CS of cataract patients is measured at high spatial frequencies, it is found to correlate well with VA and is therefore duplicating information. In cataract clinical trials, it is the lower spatial frequency CS measurements that are the most appropriate.

The cataract patient finds it difficult to distinguish relatively large objects (low spatial frequency) of low contrast from that of their surroundings, although high spatial frequency objects of high contrast may be quite easily seen [15]. This is illustrated in Figure 4.5 where the normal appearance is depicted in Figure 4.5(a). In the presence of cortical cataract (Figure 4.5(b)), the name of the public house (higher contrast and spatial frequency) remains visible, although the seated person in dull clothing (lower contrast and spatial frequency) is not so well distinguished.

Since cataract patients have difficulty in perceiving low contrast objects, their ability to drive in misty or foggy conditions is certainly questionable. Indeed, the contrast-lowering effect of mist, fog and surface water thrown up by preceding vehicles is likely to reduce the visual performance of the patient to levels below those of the legal driving standards.

It has also been demonstrated that when the cataract is uniocular, the binocular CS is reduced at high spatial frequencies by binocular inhibition [16]. Thus, the vision of these patients is more affected than measurements on the better eye alone would indicate.

There are many CS charts available to optometrists in clinical practice (see Chapter 5). These include the Pelli–Robson Chart and the Cambridge low-contrast gratings test. They are designed to give a relatively rapid assessment of a patient's visual function whilst being inexpensive and easy to use.

4.3.5 Glare

As mentioned above, cataract causes light to be scattered towards the retina (forward scattered light) and, in turn, this causes glare. The closer a light source is to the object of regard, the greater the glare and the more poorly perceived is the object. Cataract ranks high in the list of conditions causing poor vision at dusk or at night. In photopic conditions, when the pupil is constricted, the effect of early cortical cataract in scattering light is minimized. However, if the pupil dilates normally, there is a marked influence in mesopic conditions. Patients with early cortical cataract find difficulty in driving at night although their photopic VA may be quite satisfactory.

Night time driving is the most commonly reported situation which involves the problem of glare. Figure 4.6(a) is a view through a normal eye of a street scene at night. Figure 4.6(b) is the same scene viewed through a simulated cortical cataract. It is quite obvious that it is impossible for the cataract patient to cross the road with any safety. Most patients in the age range of 50–60 years who drive report that they are dazzled by other car headlights at night. Often, they complain that other road users no longer dip their headlights. However, at the age of 50–60 years the normal crystalline lens causes significant light scatter, thus leading to glare and reduced visual performance of the middle-aged driver.

In Chapter 5 the techniques of glare testing will be discussed. Briefly, glare has a relatively weak effect at high contrast and is most appropriately measured with a standardized glare source surrounding a contrast sensitivity test display [15]. Clinical instruments to measure glare, such as the brightness acuity tester (BAT), are commercially available (see Chapter 5). However, a simple and effective assessment of glare in cataract can be obtained by asking the patient to read a Snellen chart, whilst a pen torch positioned 30 cm away, is directed into the eye under investigation. A normal eye will be unaffected but the eye with cataract is likely to suffer reduced performance when the pen torch is used.

Opacities that do not lie within the pupillary boundary can also cause glare if they receive light from oblique rays. This light is scattered within the eye thus causing glare. Bright objects that are in the peripheral field, such as a reading lamp, can be troublesome to the cataract patient.

4.3.6 Colour shift

The normal ageing lens exhibits a progressive increase in absorption of the blue end of the spectrum [17,18], and the effect of cataract formation, especially nuclear, further increases this absorption. Nuclear cataract has two quite distinct components: nuclear white scatter and nuclear brunescence. The white scatter can often be seen with the slit lamp (see Figure 4.2(b)). The nuclear brunescence is a brown pigmentation which absorbs and can colour the nucleus from amber to black. The nuclear brunescence is best seen by observing the colour of the slit lamp beam focused on the posterior capsule of the crystalline lens, when viewed in optical section. These two features of the nuclear cataract can be seen independently but are more commonly seen in combination.

The attenuation of light at the blue end of the spectrum can cause a tritanomalous condition. This slow shift in colour perception with age is not often noticed by the patient. However, famous classical oil painters have been known to have a 'blue period' during their later years. This is thought to be attributed to the decrease in blue light reaching the retina with advancing age, so the painter feels the need to add more blue to the picture for it to have the same visual effect.

Figure 4.7 shows four photographs of Durham Cathedral. Figure 4.7(a) simulates the view through a normal healthy lens, and Figure 4.7(b) is the same scene viewed through a simulated cortical cataract. The effect of a colour shift caused by nuclear brunescence is depicted in Figure 4.7(c). The more usual situation of coexisting brunescence and white scatter is shown in Figure 4.7(d). With the sudden removal of the crystalline lens during cataract surgery, wavelengths from the blue end of the spectrum reach the retina in greater quantities. The return to a more normal retinal spectral distribution can give rise to symptoms including heightened colour perception. The simple deduction that vision should appear more blue is not always borne out in the patient's report. Blue, red, green or yellow vision have all been described, as have other changes in colour vision. After cataract extraction, the novel depth and brightness of the colours seen through the lens implant are often far more amazing to the patient than the improvement in acuity.

4.3.7 Reduced light transmission

With advancing age, the normal crystalline lens increases in thickness and this causes the lens to transmit progressively less light [17,18]. At the same time, the lens loses transparency as a result of increased light scatter [19] and absorption [20]. An additional factor in reduced retinal illumination with age is the inability of the ageing pupil to dilate in poor light. Even the ageing human retina has a tremendous ability to change its sensitivity to light and this is usually more than adequate to compensate for the reduced lens transmission. In poor light, however, the absorption by the cataract becomes critical. Much less light reaches the retina and vision is reduced. Other visual effects of cataract, already described, are often exaggerated in

poor light and these can combine to reduce vision.

On the whole, therefore, cataract patients have better vision in good, rather than poor, illumination. However, if the cataract is small in extent and is placed on the visual axis, the vision of the patient is improved if the pupil is allowed to dilate.

4.3.8 Field loss

The visual field can be affected by cataract. If the opacity is moderate to large, it can cast a shadow on the retina thus causing a peripheral field defect. If cataract and glaucoma coexist, then this often creates a problem in differential diagnosis. In particular, the reduced light transmission caused by cataract can cause an established glaucomatous field defect to apparently increase as the cataract progresses, when the field is tested with quantitative perimetry [21,22]. However, this effect can be reversed if the illumination of the test stimulus is increased. Nevertheless, a degree of uncertainty as to what is actually happening at the retinal level still remains.

4.3.9 Visual acuity reduction

VA measurement gives a poor assessment of a patient's visual performance and that is why it is dealt with last in this list of the subjective effects of cataract.

As outlined above, the measurement of VA in the clinical situation, under ideal conditions, does not relate to the conditions of the real world. The Snellen letters, for example, are of very high contrast (almost 100%) and the examination room is usually free from glare sources. Patients will very rarely experience such good visual conditions in their everyday life. For example, newspaper print possesses a contrast well below 100%. Also, it has been found that if VAs are measured out of doors, a lower standard is achieved [23].

The Snellen value of 6/12 is commonly regarded as approximating to the minimal UK visual driving standard. However, in poor visibility conditions, in combination with other car headlights, the patient with cataract would be

unlikely to meet the standard. Thus, VA measurement in a clinical situation tends to overestimate the patient's visual ability [9].

4.4 Refraction and optical management

Refraction is fundamental to the management of cataract. This section will not attempt to painstakingly explain each step of the refraction process. However, certain important aspects of refraction which are particularly significant when dealing with cataract patients will be given special consideration.

Retinoscopy may be difficult or even impossible, depending upon the extent of the cataract. A poor retinal reflex is the usual problem and, in the case of moderate to large degrees of cataract, retinoscopy is likely to be of little value, except perhaps to give an early indication of the cataract type and severity. Reducing the working distance for retinoscopy may increase the brightness of the retinal reflex but this is unlikely to improve its quality significantly. In addition, the small working distance can lead to poorer precision. In some cases, it can be more accurate and less time-consuming not to perform retinoscopy but to concentrate on subjective refraction.

In order to predict improvement in vision and patient satisfaction after dispensing, refraction should be conducted under conditions which best resemble those of the normal living and working conditions of the patient. This may, however, be very difficult to achieve. Nevertheless, the clinician should guard against falling into the trap of thinking that an acuity improvement of only a few letters, when measured under ideal visual conditions in the clinic, will be reflected by a significant visual improvement in everyday life.

The development of a myopic shift is common in the progression of nuclear cataract (see Section 4.3.1). This serves to decrease hypermetropia. The low myopic or emmetropic patient is likely to find that the myopic shift causes their distance vision to worsen whilst at the same time their near vision without spectacles improves.

As mentioned in Section 4.3.3, astigmatic changes in refraction are common in cataract and often a small change in the cylindrical power and axis of the spectacle lens can significantly improve the patient's VA.

Owing to the dynamic nature of cataract, the change in refractive error cannot always be predicted with any certainty. The unpredictability may lead to anisometropic problems which will require careful consideration when prescribing an optical correction.

4.5 Illumination control

Cataract causes absorption, reflection and diffusion of light, all of which serve to reduce retinal illumination (see Section 4.3.7) which in turn leads to a poor retinal image. Increasing the illumination of visual tasks does not always improve the quality of the retinal image. Increasing the illumination reduces the pupil size which decreases the amount of light reaching the retina. In addition, bright light sources in the visual field cause disability glare, which further degrades the retinal image (see Sections 4.3.4 and 4.3.5). If the amount of light entering the eye is too great for a particular visual task, it will have a contrast lowering effect. In this respect, it is important to control the illumination to suit individual needs, rather than by simply using maximum illumination.

4.5.1 Reading lamps

It is a good practice to tell patients that with increasing age there is a need for increased illumination on near-visual tasks. Many patients may be aware of this but do not know how to control their near-vision illumination. It is best to instruct the patient to use a directable reading lamp for near tasks. With this, the light can be directed on to the area of interest, rather than simply causing a general increase in brightness. The lamp should be situated so that the light shines from behind and above the patient's shoulder on to the task, without the lamp or shade being visible to the patient. The near task should be evenly illuminated and free of shadows. In general, a 40–60 W bulb in a reading lamp is adequate for most near tasks. This will produce an illumination of 1000 lux which is the recommended illuminance for fine close work [24].

4.5.2 Typoscope

This is an inexpensive instrument which can easily be made and which often yields significant benefits for the cataract patient. It is a black piece of card with a rectangle cut in its centre which extends about 2 cm vertically and 1 or 2 columns of print horizontally (Figure 4.8). It should be placed flat on the page and moved along the lines of the passage being read. The black card reduces the amount of light reflected into the patient's eyes whilst allowing the print to be adequately illuminated.

4.5.3 Shades

A peaked cap or eye shade is useful in preventing light from above the patient's head entering the eye and causing glare. They are especially useful to the patient in preventing ceiling lights from becoming glare sources and when walking about in bright sunlight.

4.5.4 Tinted lenses

Argument still exists over the value of tinted lenses for cataract patients. Some manufacturers produce lenses which are photochromic and which absorb ultraviolet and the visible blue end of the spectrum. It is possible that such lenses reduce light scatter for the patient. However, there is still no significant evidence that these lenses have any benefit over other types of tint for cataract patients.

Each patient should be treated as an individual case. If the cataract is on the visual axis, the patient will probably benefit from wearing a dark tint in bright conditions, since this will help to prevent the pupil from constricting fully and will reduce the problem of the cataract filling the pupillary area. However, if the cataract is peripheral, the patient may have better vision in bright conditions when the pupil is allowed to constrict. Under such circumstances, the wearing of a tint to help the pupil to dilate would be detrimental. In any case, patients are best advised to avoid wearing tinted lenses in poor light as this reduces contrast and may result in accidents.

4.5.5 Mydriasis

In the past a mydriatic drug has been used for patients with cataract on the visual axis. If this therapy is undertaken, it has to be on a long-term basis in order to keep the pupil dilated and to increase the amount of light entering the eye around the cataract. Although this can significantly improve the acuity of the patient, it is not often used nowadays because of the possibility of closed-angle glaucoma. There is also the risk of drug-induced side effects.

4.6 Referral

Specific referral criteria for an ophthalmological opinion are dealt with elsewhere (see Chapter 7). Only general points that require consideration are discussed here.

There are still those optometrists who base the timing of their referral solely on the level of the VA of the patient. It must be said that some ophthalmologists continue to have this as a basis for referral too. This may be due to the pressure of surgical waiting lists. Nevertheless, the majority of ophthalmologists seem to want optometrists to use the criterion of functional need of the patient, rather than VA level, for referral. In other words, the optometrist must make a clinical decision as to the extent of the effect of the cataract upon the life style of the individual patient. For example, a taxi driver will require relatively good acuity, and surgery may be necessary at an earlier stage than for a more sedentary patient.

It is important for optometrists and ophthalmologists who work in the same geographical region to communicate with each other for several reasons. Firstly, the basis of when to refer patients can be determined, and secondly, the optometrist gains information on the surgical procedures from the ophthalmologist. Thus, the optometrist will be aware of the likelihood of inpatient or outpatient surgery, the type of aphakic correction favoured by the ophthalmologists, and the time required for recovery. A patient who requires referral can then be given a more comprehensive picture of what may happen after the consultation.

4.7 Patient education

If a patient is told that a cataract exists in one or both eyes, then she or he should be given an explanation in layman's terms of the nature of the cataract, its location, how it may affect VA and an indication of its rate of progression. The use of model eyes, along with patient leaflets and handouts with illustrations, is a good way of giving the patient correct information. It is important to emphasize that, although cataract progression is likely to cause visual deterioration, it poses no serious threat to general or ocular health. Also, the patient is usually reassured to know that, although surgery is required, in most cases the VA can be restored to normal or near-normal levels.

4.8 Management according to cataract type

4.8.1 Bilateral congenital cataract

The management of bilateral congenital cataract depends on the degree to which the lens opacity is interfering with retinal image formation and the presence of other ocular or systemic disease. If the opacity is small, management should be directed to the treatment of any other ocular abnormalities, such as significant refractive error or strabismic amblyopia. However, if the opacity is more dense and central, the degree to which this affects vision is difficult to assess. Some children with central opacity may benefit from mydriatics to allow more peripheral light rays to reach the retina. In more severe cases of cataract, when the fovea is deprived of a clear image, the child runs the risk of developing amblyopia which makes the necessity for cataract surgery more pressing. An indication that significant visual handicap is present is the development of pendular nystagmus. Treatment for such severe cases is usually bilateral cataract extraction within the first few weeks of life. Obviously, postoperative visual correction is vital, otherwise amblyopia will develop.

4.8.2 Unilateral congenital cataract

An otherwise healthy eye with a moderately dense congenital cataract has a very poor prognosis for good vision when the fellow eye is normal. The patient will always use the better eye in preference to the cataractous eye, which is likely to become amblyopic in spite of early surgery and good refractive correction. Nevertheless, the optometrist should always refer unilateral congenital cataract cases for an ophthalmological opinion.

4.8.3 Acquired cataract in children

The principles of management of bilateral acquired cataract are the same as for bilateral congenital cataract. The examination of such patients involves an investigation for underlying metabolic and ocular disorders. Unilateral acquired cataract in childhood is usually a result of trauma. Provided that the eye is not other-wise significantly damaged, the best management is for the cataract to be extracted, followed by optimum refractive correction of that eye. This should be done as early as possible to prevent the development of amblyopia. However, the older the child at the time of the injury, the less chance there is of any amblyopic complication.

4.8.4 Acquired cataract in adults

An adult patient who develops cataract should be investigated for underlying pathological conditions, such as diabetes, which are known to be cataractogenic. Also, it is important to establish the extent of the visual deterioration which is due to the cataract alone, as opposed to coexisting corneal, retinal or neural disease.

Surgical treatment of bilateral cataract is usually only performed when the patient's life style is significantly affected. It is, therefore, very important for the optometrist to assess the patient's life style and related visual requirements.

Unilateral cataract in an adult is often surgically removed at an earlier stage than if it is bilateral, especially if good binocular vision is required. This is particularly the case when good binocular vision is essential for occupational or employment purposes. The usual methods of refractive correction of a unilateral aphake are to use an intraocular lens implant (IOL) or less commonly a contact lens. The IOL gives better equalization of image sizes between the two eyes.

4.9 Conclusion

As the geriatric population continues to increase, optometrists can expect to examine more and more patients with cataract. Awareness of the diagnostic features of the different morphological types of cataract, knowledge of the likely progression of each type and the signs and symptoms that result will facilitate better patient management. Patient education is an important area which requires development in order for patients to be aware that, in isolation, cataract is not a serious eye disease.

Whilst cataract is progressing, the optometrist can best help the patient by performing a thorough refraction in order to detect any change in prescription. Guidance on illumination control and knowledge of when to refer for an ophthalmological opinion are important factors in ensuring that the patient receives the best possible management.

Acknowledgements

I would like to thank Mr Nicholas Phelps-Brown, Honorary Consultant to the Radcliffe Infirmary, Oxford and Consultant Ophthalmic Surgeon, Harley Street, London. The *Optician* is acknowledged for its permission to use material which has been previously published.

References

1. Miller, D. The nude in the shower phenomenon. *Survey of Ophthalmology,* **16**, 332 (1972)
2. Sparrow, J.M., Bron, A.J., Brown, N.A.P., Ayliffe, W. and Hill, A.R. The Oxford Clinical Cataract Classification and Grading System. *International Ophthalmology,* **9**, 207–225 (1986)
3. Chyalck, L.T., White, O. and Tung, W.H. Classification of human senile cataractous change by the American Co-operative Cataract research group (CCRG) method II. Staged simplification of cataract classification. *Investigative Ophthalmology and Visual Science,* **25**, 166–173 (1984)
4. Brown, N.A.P., Bron, A.J. and Sparrow, J.M. Methods for evaluation of lens changes. *International Ophthalmology,* **12**, 229–235 (1988)
5. Sparrow, J.M., Brown, N.A.P., Shun-Shin, G.A. and Bron, A.J. The Oxford modular cataract image analysis system. *Eye,* **4**, 638–648 (1990)
6. Harris, M.L., Smith, G.T.H. and Brown, N.A.P. Inter and intra observer reproducibility of the new Oxford CCD Scheimpflug camera. *Eye,* **5**, 487–490 (1991)
7. Slataper, F.J. Age norms of refraction and vision. *Archives of Ophthalmology,* **43**, 466–481 (1950)
8. Brown, N.A.P. and Hill, A.R. Cataract: the relationship between myopia and cataract morphology. *British Journal of Ophthalmology,* **71**, 405–414 (1987)
9. Hess, R. and Woo, G. Vision through cataracts. *Investigative Ophthalmology and Visual Science,* **17**, 428–435 (1978)
10. Paulsson, L.E. and Sjostrand, J. Contrast sensitivity in the presence of a glare light. *Investigative Ophthalmology and Visual Science,* **19**, 401–406 (1980)
11. Skalka, H.W. Arden grating test in evaluating 'early' posterior subcapsular cataracts. *Southern Medical Journal,* **74**, 1368–1370 (1981)
12. Koch, D.D. Glare and contrast sensitivity testing an cataract patients. *Journal of Cataract and Refractive Surgery,* **15**, 158–164 (1989)
13. Elliott, D.B., Hurst, M.A. and Weatherill, J. Comparing clinical tests of visual function in cataract with the patients perceived visual disability. *Eye,* **4**, 712–717 (1990)
14. Elliott, D.B., Gilchrist, J. and Whitaker, D. Contrast sensitivity and glare sensitivity changes with three types of cataract morphology: are these techniques necessary in a clinical evaluation of cataract? *Ophthalmic and Physiological Optics,* **9**, 25–30 (1989)
15. Elliott, D.B., Gilchrist, J., Pickwell, L.D. Sheridan, M., Weatherill, J. and Whitaker, D. The subjective assessment of cataract. *Ophthalmic and Physiological Optics,* **9**, 16–19 (1989)
16. Pardhan, S. and Gilchrist, J. The importance of measuring binocular contrast sensitivity in unilateral cataract. *Eye,* **5**, 31–35 (1991)
17. Boettener, E.A. and Wolter, J.R. Transmission of ocular media. *Investigative Ophthalmology,* **1**, 776 (1962)
18. Lerman, S. and Borkman, R.F. Spectroscopic evaluation and classification of normal ageing and cataractous lens. *Ophthalmic Research,* **8**, 335–353 (1976)
19. Smith, G.T.H., Smith, R.C., Brown, N.A.P., Bron, A.J. and Harris, M.C. Changes in light scatter and width measurements from the human cortex with age. *Eye,* **6**, 55–59 (1992)
20. Mellerio, J. Yellowing of the human lens: nuclear and cortical contributions. *Vision Research,* **27**, 1581–1587 (1987)
21. Guthauser, U. and Flammer, J. Quantifying visual field damage caused by cataract. *American Journal of Ophthalmology,* **106**, 480–484 (1988)
22. Heider, H.W., Sees, K.J. and Schnaudigel, O.E. Cataract induced visual field changes. *Klinische Monatsblatter fur Augenheilkunde,* **198**, 15–19 (1991)
23. Holladay, J.J., Prager, T.C., Trujillo, J. and Ruiz, R.S. Brightness acuity test and outdoor VA in cataract patients. *Journal of Cataract and Refractive Surgery,* **13**, 67–69 (1987)
24. Durrant, D.W. (ed.) *Interior Lighting Design,* 5th edn, Lighting Industry Federation Limited and The Electricity Council, London, pp. 58–59 (1980)

5

New clinical techniques to evaluate cataract

David B. Elliott

The only proven treatment for cataract is surgery. There is currently no effective medical treatment for cataract in either the UK or North America. Unproved treatments are offered in various European and Far East countries [1]. Nutritional, herbal and homoeopathic treatments have been advocated [2], and laboratory experiments on animals have suggested a beneficial effect of various dietary antioxidants such as certain vitamins [3]. However, this remains a relatively unused alternative treatment. Therefore, a common problem facing many clinicians is deciding when surgery is appropriate for cataract patients.

5.1 A brief history of 'when to operate'

Historians are unsure whether it was the Egyptians or the Ancient Indians who first performed cataract surgery [4,5]. The first description in the medical literature is contained in Celsus' *De re Medicina*. This is the oldest Greco–Latin medical document, after the Hippocratic writings, and appeared around AD 29. Celsus' account of what was later called 'couching' describes the creation of an opening in the capsule using a sharp needle and then dislocating the lens. A more detailed account of the procedure can be found in the writings of Paullus of Aegina (7th century AD). The treatment and preoperative assessment of cataract described in these very early writings endured without significant change, until the 18th century [4,5]. The decision

of when to operate depended upon the 'ripeness' of the cataract. Cataracts had to be a steel grey or blue colour before the operation could be successfully completed. The decision of when to operate also seems to have depended on the patient's level of vision. When a cataract patient had no light perception, the operations were frequently unsuccessful because of underlying ocular disease. Lens extraction came in the 18th century and is accredited to the Frenchman Jacques Daviel (1693–1762). The detailed case histories of the 18th century surgeons, such as Daviel [4] and Richter [6], make fascinating reading. Treatment included blooding and purging with diets of gruel and the oil of sweet almonds. The decision of when to operate remained dependent on the ripeness of the cataract and whether the patient could see light.

Surgery was further improved with the introduction of anaesthesia and Lister's antisepsis in the middle and late 19th century [5]. Although Helmholtz's invention of the ophthalmoscope in 1850 revolutionized the general practice of ophthalmology, it had little impact on cataract surgery. Surgeons continued to wait for cataracts to ripen before performing extraction until as late as the early 1900s [7]. In such situations, of course, viewing the retina is not possible. Various artificial ripening techniques were devised to quicken up the process. If operated upon before this time, the lens was not always removed cleanly because of the stickiness of the unripe cortex. This led to possible ocular irritation and 'after-cataract'. Improved techniques for the removal of persisting cortical remnants and after-cataract, along with the introduction of intracapsular extraction, resulted in more immature cataracts being extracted. The decision of when to operate became more dependent on the influence of the cataract on the patient's ability to function normally. Unilateral and second eye cataract extractions increased after the invention of the intraocular implant introduced by Harold Ridley at St Thomas' Hospital, London, in 1949. Ridley had seen many ocular injuries caused by the shattering of Spitfire canopies during World War II [8]. He discovered that the imbedded plastic material did not produce any ocular reaction. The first recorded suggestion of using an optical aid (a magnifying glass) implanted in the eye, was made in the 18th century by Giacomo Casanova [8]. He is perhaps best remembered for some of his other accomplishments!

The ever increasing improvements in cataract surgery and intraocular lens design changed patients' attitudes towards the operation. This, coupled with an increased need for better vision in the elderly, has resulted in a growing number of patients being operated on at an earlier stage of cataract development. By the 1970s, the decision to extract an uncomplicated age-related cataract was generally based on two factors:

(a) whether the diminished vision was interfering with the patient's ability to function in their desired life style;
(b) whether any other ocular disease was present [9].

These criteria were obviously open to wide interpretation. A general guideline of 6/18 visual acuity (VA) (20/60 in North America) was often used as a suitable indicator of visual loss, below which cataract should be extracted [9].

5.2 Reliable VA measurements

Although entrenched as the standard in vision assessment, the conventional Snellen chart has not changed a great deal since Snellen's Optotypes were introduced in 1862 [10]. Several LogMAR VA charts [11–14] are now available, based on the original Bailey–Lovie chart [11] (Figure 5.1). They have several advantages over the traditional Snellen charts:

(a) the same number of letters on every line;

(b) a logarithmic progression in size from 1 line to the next. This scale of progression provides equal perceptual steps;
(c) the above allows the use of a letter by letter scoring system, which has been shown to provide high test–retest reliability.

LogMAR VA charts have quickly become the standard for clinical research because of the inaccuracy of Snellen charts at reduced VA levels, where Snellen charts generally have only one or two letters. LogMAR charts are also widely used in low vision clinics and it is hoped they will find more widespread use in general clinical practice.

5.3 The inadequacy of VA

Using a VA of 6/18 as a guideline for cataract extraction has been shown to be inadequate in a significant number of cases (even when VA is measured accurately using a logMAR chart). Some sedentary patients who only wish to read are perfectly content with VAs much worse than 6/18. More importantly, many clinicians have reported seeing patients who retain much better VA than 6/18, yet report significant visual problems [9,15–22]. Presumably, some aspect of vision, which is not measured by VA, is impaired in some cataract patients. It has been suggested that contrast sensitivity (CS) and disability glare scores provide additional information about visual disability in cataract. Low spatial frequency CS and glare test scores have been shown not to correlate with VA. Significant reductions in CS and increases in glare scores have been found in cataract patients with minimally impaired VA [15–22]. The rationale behind CS and glare testing of cataractous patients is that scores will be poor in those who possess reasonable VA yet complain of significant visual problems.

5.4 Contrast sensitivity: what does it measure?

CS measurements traditionally involve determinations of the minimum contrast required to detect a vertical sine-wave grating of a certain thickness (spatial frequency). The minimum contrast is called the contrast threshold, and CS is defined as the reciprocal of the contrast threshold. A plot of CS over a range of spatial

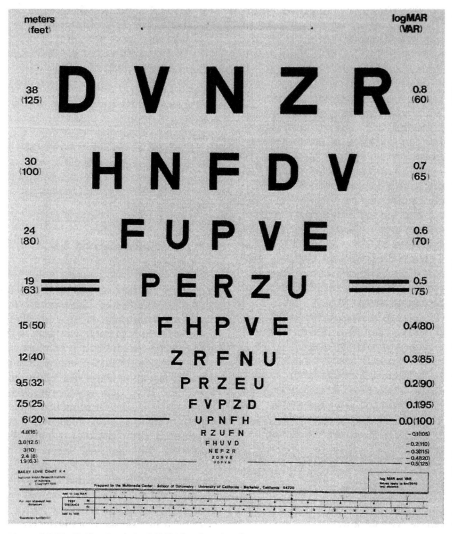

Figure 5.1 The Bailey–Lovie logMAR visual acuity chart.

frequencies gives the contrast sensitivity function (CSF). A normal photopic CSF is shown in Figure 5.2. This illustrates a bell shaped curve, with a clear peak at intermediate spatial frequencies, around 2–6 cycles/degree (c/deg). This peak is often used to divide the CSF into low, intermediate and high spatial frequencies. The CSF shows a rapid fall off in sensitivity at higher spatial frequencies and a more gradual fall at lower frequencies. The point where the CSF cuts the *x*-axis indicates the finest pattern which is just detectable at maximum contrast which theoretically corresponds to the VA. VA has been shown to be highly correlated with the high spatial frequency portion of the CS curve

[23–26]. These high spatial frequency responses provide little or no information regarding the low and intermediate frequencies [23–28].

5.5 Light scatter in cataract

Visual loss in cataract is mainly due to increased intraocular light scatter [29]. Figure 5.3 shows how this produces a veiling luminance which reduces the contrast of the retinal image.

Hess and Woo's classic paper [30] on CS in unilateral cataract indicated that cataract preferentially reduces high-frequency CS. They found less CS loss at low frequencies and

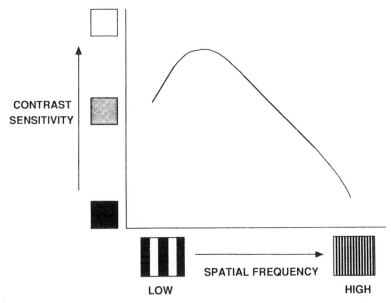

Figure 5.2 The typical shape of a contrast sensitivity function (CSF) for a subject with normal healthy eyes.

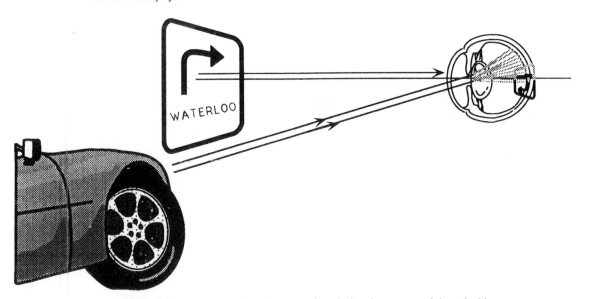

Figure 5.3 Schematic representation of the effects of a glare source in reducing the contrast of the retinal image.

suggested this was because cataract produces only slight scatter immediately around the direction of the refracted rays. Such narrow-angle light scatter would preferentially affect the contrast of fine gratings. As VA measurements give an indication of high spatial frequencies, VA can be used to assess the effect of narrow-angle light scatter on a cataract patient's vision [30,31]. Hess and Woo [30] also found a few patients who showed reduced CS at low spatial frequencies, which was unrelated to their VA. They suggested that light must have been scattered over a much wider angle to affect such large gratings.

These patterns of CS loss have been confirmed by several later studies [31,32,33]. Consider the two patients whose binocular CS curves are displayed in Figure 5.4 where the

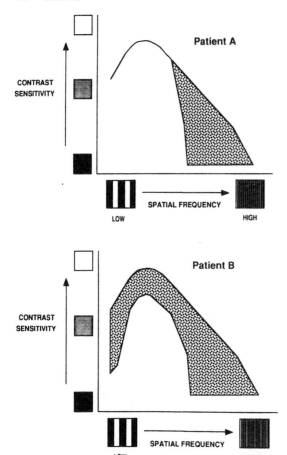

Figure 5.4 The loss (shaded areas) in contrast sensitivity (CS) of two hypothetical patients A and B. Both have the same visual acuity of about 6/12. Patient A has CS loss only at high spatial frequencies, while patient B has CS loss at all spatial frequencies.

shaded areas represent the areas of visual loss. Both have 6/12 binocular VA, indicated by both CSFs cutting the *x*-axis at the same point. Patient A has CS loss only at high spatial frequencies. Patient B, however, has loss over the whole spatial frequency curve. Therefore, although the patients have the same VA, their visual impairments differ. Research has shown that, in patients with cataract and other ocular diseases, low-frequency CS is a better measure of perceived visual disability than VA [34–36]. When evaluating the vision of a cataract patient, VA assesses the effect of narrow-angle light scatter. In addition, an evaluation of wide-angle light scatter is needed [37]. This can be obtained using low spatial frequency CS measurements [38] or disability glare tests [37] (see section 5.8).

5.6 Clinical CS tests

Low-contrast letter charts are not, contrary to popular opinion, a recent phenomenon; 70 years ago it was possible to purchase George Young's contrast sensitivity test apparatus from J. Weiss of London. Even earlier, in 1889, a Swedish ophthalmologist had described low-contrast letter charts. We are currently improving our understanding of how measurements of CS can usefully support traditional VA measurements and recognizing in which patients CS measurements are likely to be most useful [14]. The most widely available charts are the Vistech CS system [39], the Bailey–Lovie [11], Regan low-contrast acuity charts [14] and the Pelli–Robson letter CS chart [24].

With the introduction of these charts, CS is becoming more widely used in clinical practice. For example, in a recent survey of ophthalmologists of the American Society of Cataract and Refractive Surgery, 29% of respondents were using CS as part of their routine assessment of cataract [40]. Most of these were using the Vistech 6500 CS system.

5.6.1 The Vistech CS system

The Vistech CS system can be used at either distance (VCTS 6500) or near (VCTS 6000). Five spatial frequencies can be tested at 1.5, 3, 6, 12 and 18 c/deg. Several studies have shown that these charts have poor test–retest reliability [25,41–44]. In addition, from a clinical viewpoint, it seems unnecessary to measure the whole CS curve to evaluate cataract. All that is needed is an accurate VA measurement and an assessment of CS at low spatial frequencies [22,25,26,31].

5.6.2 The Pelli–Robson chart

This is an 86 × 63 cm chart which is hung 1 m from the patient's eye and is shown in Figure 5.5. The chart consists of 16 triplets of 4.9 × 4.9 cm letters. The chart gives an indication of CS just below the peak of the curve at 0.5–2 c/deg. Within each triplet, the letters have the same contrast and the contrast in each successive triplet decreases by a factor of 0.15 log units. The patient is asked to read as far down the chart as they can. One disadvantage of the chart is that scores will vary depending on the time the patient is allowed to study letters

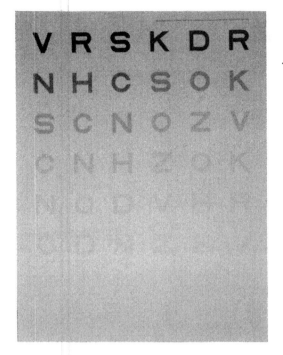

Figure 5.5 The Pelli–Robson chart. (Reproduced with permission of Clement Clarke Inc., Columbus, Ohio, USA.)

near threshold [26]. Scores tend to be at least 0.15 log units lower if a patient is not given sufficient time. The letter C is often called as an O and this can be taken as a correct call [45]. A log CS score is determined by subtracting 0.05 log units for each letter incorrectly called from the log CS value of the last triplet in which any letter is seen. This scoring rule has been shown to provide better test–retest reliability than the original [46].

5.6.3 Bailey–Lovie charts

A 10% contrast Bailey–Lovie logMAR chart [47] is commercially available (10% Michelson contrast corresponds to 18% Weber contrast). Michelson contrast is defined as:

$$\frac{L_{max} - L_{min}}{L_{max} + L_{min}}$$

This is generally used when calculating contrast for sine-wave gratings. L_{max} and L_{min} are the respective luminances of the light and dark bars of the grating.

Weber contrast is defined as:

$$\frac{L_b - L_t}{L_b}$$

It is generally used when calculating the contrast of letters or other targets. L_b and L_t are the respective luminances of the background and the target.

5.6.4 The Regan charts

These are logMAR acuity charts of varying contrast, with a working distance of 3 m. In addition to the traditional high-contrast chart (Weber contrast 96%), Regan charts of 50%, 25%, 11% and 4% are available [14]. The 96% and 11% chart are the most useful for cataract evaluations [38,48]. When using the Regan charts to measure disability glare in cataracts, the 25% chart should be used [38,48]. The Regan charts are very similar in design to the Bailey–Lovie. They differ slightly in that the letters use a different font configuration and there are eight letters per acuity row rather than five. In addition, the Regan charts use 5×5 Sloan letters whereas the Bailey–Lovie uses 4×5 British Standard (BS 4274) letters (Figure 5.6).

The Pelli–Robson chart measures the contrast threshold of letters of a fixed size. The Regan and Bailey–Lovie charts, however, measure the smallest letter that can be resolved at a fixed contrast. These charts measure low contrast acuity, not CS (Figure 5.7). If only the large letters at the top of the chart can be seen, the score gives an indication of CS at intermediate spatial frequencies. If a patient can see the small letters at the bottom of the chart, the score gives an indication of higher spatial frequency performance.

All letter charts have the advantage of being familiar to both clinician and patient. The three letter charts described above all provide reliable, simple and quick measurements of CS or acuity [38]. The Pelli–Robson chart is probably the most effective CS chart to use with cataract patients as it measures low spatial frequency CS and can be used to complement traditional VA measurements [22,38,49].

5.7 Disadvantages of measuring CS in cataract

The major disadvantage of using CS to evaluate visual function in cataract is that, like VA loss, CS loss is not specific to cataract [50]. If a patient has both cataract and other ocular

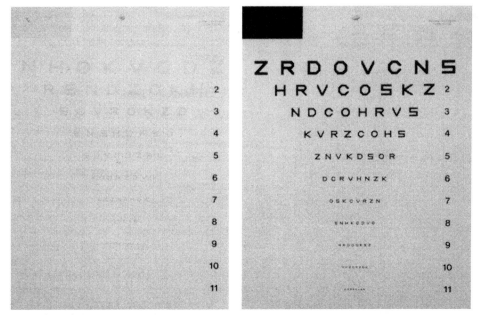

Figure 5.6 The Regan 25% and 96% contrast logMAR charts. (Reproduced with permission of Dr David Regan, University of York, Canada.)

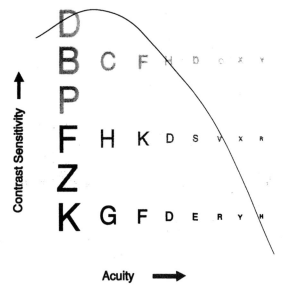

Figure 5.7 A schematic representation of the difference between letter contrast sensitivity measurements (e.g. Pelli–Robson charts) and low-contrast acuity measurements (e.g. Bailey–Lovie, Regan).

pathology, the clinician does not know how much of the CS (or VA) loss is due to the cataract.

Disability glare tests provide a more sensitive assessment of wide-angle light scatter than clinical CS tests [38].

5.8 Disability glare

The vision of a cataract patient is reduced most in glare or bright light conditions. Many patients, for example, have difficulty seeing objects against oncoming car headlights. Indeed, cataract patients often stop driving at night for this reason. Looking through a dirty windscreen in bright sunlight, or when driving at night, seems to be a very useful way of simulating the effect of cataract on vision (Figure 5.3). This demonstrates the inadequacy of assessing the visual performance of cataract patients by using VA measurements taken in the typical no-glare low-light examination room.

Lucretius provided an early description of glare nearly 2000 years ago: 'Bright things the eyes eschew and shun to look upon; the sun even blinds them, if you persist in turning towards it because its power is great and idols are borne through the clear air with great downward force and strike the eyes and disorder their fastenings'. There are two main types of glare: discomfort glare and disability glare. The latter reduces visual performance without necessarily causing discomfort. A fine example of the value of glare testing in cataract was reported by Rubin in 1972 [15]. A healthy 45-year-old prison guard complaining of a gradual decrease in his vision over the previous year was seen. This only occurred in bright sunlight, as when guarding prisoners working outside. Before his visit, his loss of vision had been so great as to allow two convicts to escape! His VAs were recorded as 6/6 in both eyes. A more careful check found VAs of 6/120 in bright light levels and slit-lamp examination revealed small posterior subcapsular cataracts.

5.9 Disability glare tests

Disability glare tests measure the reduction in a patient's visual performance due to a glare source. The light from the glare source is scattered by the cataract. As most disability glare tests use peripherally placed glare sources, the tests measure wide-angle light scatter [37]. Before 1983, when the Miller–Nadler glare tester was commercially released, clinical methods of measuring disability glare were limited. They involved measuring VA under glare conditions, such as when the chart is placed in front of a window, against the incoming light [9]. Another method was to direct the light from a penlight into the patient's eye at an angle of 15–30° from 30–45 cm [51]. These tests are simple, quick and inexpensive and continue to be used [51]. The most recently developed disability glare tests measure CS or low-contrast acuity under glare conditions. In the previously mentioned survey of American ophthalmologists, 65% stated they were routinely using CS and/or glare testing to evaluate visual function in cataract [40]. The most commonly used disability glare tests were the Miller–Nadler glare tester and the brightness acuity tester (BAT).

5.9.1 The Miller–Nadler glare tester

This was first introduced in 1972 [52] but found little clinical acceptance until reappearing in a slightly revised format in 1983 [19]. It consists of a modified slide projector with the slides presenting a series of randomly oriented Landolt rings of progressively reduced contrast (80% to 2.5%). They are surrounded by a broad glare source of constant luminance. The working distance is 40 cm. The endpoint of the test is recorded as the last correctly identified slide. It has reasonable test–retest reliability but is not sensitive to small cataractous changes because of its large step sizes (in log CS terms) at low

contrast levels [38]. Although the slides can still be purchased from Titmus Optical, the glare tester is not commercially available at the moment.

5.9.2 The brightness acuity tester (BAT)

This is a hand-held instrument which consists of a white hemispherical bowl, situated on top of a 16 cm handle [20] (Figure 5.8). The hemisphere is held over the eye and diffusely illuminated by a hidden light source. This illuminates the entire peripheral field. The patient is asked to read a chart through a small aperture in the bowl. It can be used with CS and low contrast acuity charts and with conventional high contrast VA charts. Low contrast charts provide a more sensitive measure of contrast loss [22,38,53]. Measuring traditional high-contrast VA with the BAT, however, has the advantage that the score is universally understood. The medium intensity setting of the BAT is recommended, since many early cataract patients cannot see

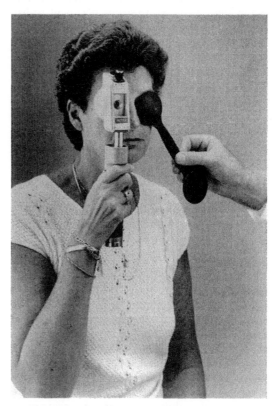

Figure 5.8 The brightness acuity tester (BAT). (Reproduced with permission of Mentor O & O Inc., Norwell, Massachusetts, USA.)

anything on the charts when the high setting is used. For this reason, the Regan 25% chart is preferred to the 11% chart when used with the BAT [38,48].

5.9.3 The Vistech MCT8000

This is an automated tabletop instrument, which uses the same targets and measurement method as the Vistech 6500. A console controls target presentation, luminance and glare source positioning. The unit allows measurement of CS at 1.5, 3, 6, 12 and 18 c/deg under night time (3.5 cd m^{-2}) and day time (137 cd m^{-2}) luminance conditions, with or without a central or peripheral glare source. The instrument provides much superfluous information and its test–retest reliability is poor [33,38].

A major problem in writing about new commercially available equipment is that it need not stay on the market for very long. In a review of glare tests published in 1991 [51], two of the five instruments listed (the Miller–Nadler and Optec glare testers) are not commercially available in 1992. It therefore seems pertinent to list the design features in a CS or glare test which are thought to be desirable. The reason that letter charts are more reliable and discriminative than the Vistech, for example, is because of their test design. The American Academy of Ophthalmology report [50] on CS and disability glare proposed the following three design principles for clinical tests:

(a)   The test should use a forced-choice psychophysical method.
(b)   Test targets should follow a uniform logarithmic progression. This scale of progression provides equal perceptual steps.
(c)   Several trials should be used at each level of acuity or contrast.

The Pelli–Robson, Regan and Bailey–Lovie tests are consistent with these three principles of test design, whereas the Vistech system possesses none. The Miller–Nadler tester uses a forced-choice method but does not incorporate design principles (b) and (c). As a consequence, the step sizes at low contrast levels are large and are the probable cause of its poorer discriminative ability [38]. The geometry and intensity of the glare source appear to be of less importance than the above chart design principles. Point glare sources are generally discouraged because of retinal adaptation problems [52].

5.10 How to use disability glare scores

Disability glare scores can be taken as either the level of CS or acuity under glare conditions or the difference in CS or acuity due to the glare source, where the difference is the score achieved in the absence of a glare source minus the score when the glare source is present. The disadvantage of the first measure, is that it is still dependent on both the cataract and the neural system [50]. The disadvantage of the second measure is that it loses sensitivity because it discards the information provided by the loss in CS or acuity without glare [38,54]. Variability is also compounded, as two measurements are used to calculate the score. CS and disability glare tests are only used to assess cataract patients with good VA. Therefore, it is generally possible to obtain an ophthalmoscopic view of the fundus and possibly an assessment of central visual fields. If such patients appear to have normal neural function, then the level of CS or acuity, in the presence of glare, should be used to help evaluate visual loss. Since glare sources enhance the effect of the cataract's light scatter, CS or acuity with glare scores are more sensitive measures of cataract than CS or acuity alone. This is most reliably measured using the BAT with any of the Pelli–Robson or low- and high-contrast charts [38].

When early cataract and neural abnormality are in combination, the difference in CS or acuity due to the glare source should be used [38,50,54]. Tests that evaluate neural function behind the cataract should also be used with these patients. These tests are discussed in Chapter 6. The Pelli–Robson chart already provides an assessment of wide-angle light scatter without the glare source. Further measurements using the BAT only slightly increase the efficacy of the test [38,54]. When an assessment of disability glare is needed in a cataract patient with neural abnormality, the low- or high-contrast VA charts with the BAT are preferred. Without glare, they predominantly assess narrow angle light scatter, so the reduction in acuity due to the glare source reflects wide-angle light scatter only [38].

5.11 Normal data collection

Clinicians differ in the values they obtain using any test that requires patient subjective responses [26]. Normative data provided with a chart may not compare well with data a clinician would acquire from patients with normal vision. It is advisable for clinicians to obtain their own normative data. This provides good experience with the chart and the scoring system. Measurements should be collected from patients of each decade since age can possibly affect scores. Taking a mean for each decade will give an average score and the mean minus 2 standard deviations provides a lower limit which could be accepted as being normal.

5.12 Future research

The rationale behind CS and glare testing is that CS is low in the presence of a glare source in cataract patients with reasonable VA, who complain of significant visual problems. This has yet to be proven. Most of the evidence is anecdotal, in the form of case reports [15,22,55]. Perceived visual disability in cataract has been shown to be more correlated with CS and CS with glare than VA [21,36]. Interestingly, binocular CS correlated best of all with perceived visual disability in cataract [36]. This is perhaps not surprising since most people perceive binocularly but most clinical tests are measured monocularly. With VA measures, binocular scores correlate highly with 'best' eye scores [56]. This casts some doubt on the value of binocular VA measurement. Binocular CS measurements, however, are affected by the monocular CS of both eyes [32,56]. Where the CS is equal in both eyes, the binocular CS is about 42% greater than the best monocular response because of binocular summation. In patients who have differences in CS between the two eyes, binocular summation is less than 42%. In some cases binocular CS can even be less than the best monocular response [32,56]. This has been called binocular inhibition. The same pattern occurs with CS levels in the presence of glare. Perhaps those patients who complain of their bad eye affecting the vision of their good eye actually have binocular inhibition of CS. The value of binocular measurements of both CS and disability glare in cataract patients (and others) needs to be determined by further research.

5.13 Other new techniques to evaluate cataract

5.13.1 Interzeag Opacity Lensmeter 701

The Opacity Lensmeter is a commercially available instrument that claims to give an accurate objective measure of light scatter from the lens [57]. The instrument was designed to help assess the effect of cataracts on automated visual field measurements, as well as for use in preoperative evaluation. The test basically involves illuminating the eye with a standardized red light source and measuring the amount of light scattered back. The main advantage of such a technique is that it does not require subjective responses from the patient and is independent of their neural function. Unfortunately, the Opacity Lensmeter and other techniques that use a similar method, such as Scheimpflug photography (described in Section 5.13.3.2), appear to be accurate only in assessing light scatter in the normal ageing eye and eyes affected by nuclear cataract [58,59]. Light scatter from cortical and capsular cataracts are assessed poorly, perhaps because of the irregular nature of these types of cataract. Since capsular cataracts cause the most significant visual disability, this is a major drawback in the clinical use of this instrument.

5.13.2 Cataract classification and grading systems

These basically involve classifying the cataract morphology and grading features of the cataract seen at the slit-lamp, by comparing them with standard diagrams and/or photographs. They are a less expensive more portable way of categorizing and classifying cataract than photography and are particularly useful for epidemiological studies out in the field. There are three principal systems available: the Oxford [60], LOCS III [61] and Taylor and West [62] cataract classification systems.

5.13.3 Cataract photography

Photographs provide an accurate and permanent record of the status of the cataract. The information they contain may be quantified and the photographic record can provide a baseline for evaluating change in the cataract over time. There are two principal ways of photographing cataract.

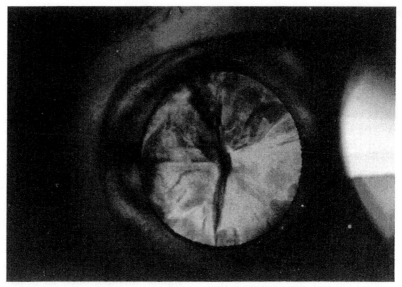

Figure 5.9 A retro-illumination photograph of cortical cataract. Photograph by M.A. Hurst, Department of Optometry, University of Bradford.

5.13.3.1 Retro-illumination photography

This shows cataracts as dark silhouettes against the background glow of the illuminated fundus, as in Figure 5.9. Fincham [63] suggested using retro-illumination photography of cataract, as the whole pupillary space can be shown in a single photograph. One disadvantage of retro-illumination photography is that the illumination of the fundus, against which the cataract is seen, is hindered by the presence of the cataract. Therefore, the technique is not as effective when very dense or extensive cataracts are photographed. Retro-illumination photographs have been taken with fundus and slit-lamp cameras [63]. Modifications have to be made to reduce the light scatter caused by direct illumination on the cornea and lens as the light journeys to the fundus. Kawara and Obazawa [64] suggested using a crossed polarizer system to remove the specular reflections from the cornea. Unfortunately, a Maltese-cross shadow can occasionally appear on photographs when this technique is used. This is caused by interference between the ordinary and extraordinary rays of corneal birefringence and also by a slight rotation of the direction of polarization of the illumination light, as it is reflected from the curved corneal surface [65,66]. Other birefringent structures, such as retrodots [67] or cholosteric crystals [68], can also impede image clarity by producing a

bright image through the polarized filters [69]. Light scatter by direct illumination of lens opacities is reduced by placing a deep orange filter in either the illumination or photographic systems [63]. This transmits the orange light from the fundus but absorbs a lot of the white light scattered by direct illumination. It also reduces the amount of corneal birefringent light scatter entering the observation system, as this light tends to be in the blue part of the spectrum [69]. Retro-illumination photography provides a useful assessment of cortical and capsular cataract but is poor at evaluating nuclear cataract [69].

5.13.3.2 Scheimpflug photography

This is a special type of slit-image photography which keeps the whole of the lens in focus by appropriately tilting the film plane [70,71]. An optical section of the lens is seen in direct illumination, with lens opacities appearing as brighter areas of greater light scatter. Slit-image photography suffers from the disadvantage that many optical sections need to be photographed to assess the whole lens. A camera which takes photographs along one section is primarily limited to the assessment of nuclear cataracts [69]. In an attempt to improve this situation, Dragomirescu *et al.* [72] developed a camera which could be rotated through 180° around the eye's optical axis. Lens section photographs could then be taken at several fixed settings, to provide a more comprehensive assessment of any cataract. Recent reports suggest that even with this adaptation, the camera is only useful for evaluating nuclear cataract [73]. Errors can occur as a result of shadows produced by lens opacities which interfere with the analysis of the posterior lens [69]. Scheimpflug photography also provides the option of measuring the thickness of the lens [69]. This may be useful as the development of cataract may affect lens thickness even in the early stages.

5.13.4 Computer image analysis

Computer image-analysis techniques can increase the usefulness of cataract photography [74]. They can be used to enhance the image, making important features more visible. They can also provide very accurate quantitative evaluation of the cataract's size, density and position [74,75]. More recently, systems have been developed which directly capture the image of the lens, using a video or charge coupled device (CCD) camera attached to the instrument. The image information is then fed directly into the computer.

5.13.5 Fluorophotometry

This technique can be used to measure fluorescent changes within the lens [76]. Lens fluorescence has been shown to increase with age, diabetes and in nuclear cataract [76] and is due to the accumulation of fluorogens within the lens. The fluorogens convert ultraviolet (UV) light into visible light. The light emitted by the fluorogens is scattered randomly and therefore can diminish the sharpness of the retinal image as a result of veiling glare [77]. This is the principal reason why UV-absorbing filters improve vision in cataractous eyes [78]. Fluorophotometry instrumentation is generally based on a traditional slit-lamp design coupled to a photomultiplier for detecting the intensity of the back scattered fluorescence.

Acknowledgements

I am grateful to Mark Bullimore (School of Optometry, Berkeley), Mary Elliott and Graham Strong (both School of Optometry, Waterloo) for valuable comments on earlier versions of this chapter and to Kathy Yang (School of Optometry, Waterloo) for the artwork. The research evaluating contrast sensitivity and disability glare tests was sponsored by the British College of Optometrists, Bausch and Lomb, the Centre for Sight Enhancement (CSE) and the Centre for Contact Lens Research (CCLR) at the University of Waterloo.

References

1. Kador, P.F. Overview of the current attempts toward the medical treatment of cataract. *Ophthalmology*, **90**, 352–364 (1983)
2. Tobe, J.H. Cataract, glaucoma and other disorders. *Prevention and Cure with Proven Natural Methods*. J.H. Tobe, St Catherines, Canada (1973)
3. Nishigori, H., Hayashi, R., Lee, J .W., Maruyama, K. and Iwatsuru, M. Preventative effect of ascorbic acid against glucocorticoid-induced cataract formation of developing chick embryos. *Experimental Eye research*, **40**, 445–451 (1985)
4. Hirschberg, J. *The History of Ophthalmology* (translated by Blodi, F. C.), Wayenburgh, Bonn (1982)
5. Grom, E. An enquiry into the history of the crystalline lens. In *Cataract and Abnormalities of the Lens* (edited by J.G. Bellows), Grune and Stratton, New York, pp. 1–28 (1975)
6. Richter, A.G. *A Treatise on the Extraction of the Cataract (1791)*, L.B. Adams, Alabama (1989)
7. May, C.H. *Diseases of the Eye*, 9th edn, W. Wood & Co., New York (1920)
8. Wilensky, J.T. *Intra-ocular Lenses*, Appleton-Century-Crofts, New York (1975)
9. Cinotti, A.A. Evaluation of indications for cataract surgery. *Ophthalmic Surgery*, **10**, 25–31 (1979)
10. Bennett, A.G. Ophthalmic test types. *British Journal of Physiological Optics*, **22**, 238–271 (1965)
11. Bailey, I.L. and Lovie, J.E. New design principles for visual acuity letter charts. *American Journal of Optometry and Physiological Optics*, **53**, 740–745 (1976)
12. Ferris, F.L., Kassof, A., Bresnick, G.H. and Bailey, I. New visual acuity charts for clinical research. *American Journal of Ophthalmology*, **94**, 91–96 (1982)
13. Strong, G. and Woo, G.C. A distance visual acuity chart incorporating some new design features. *Archives of Ophthalmology*, **103**, 44–46 (1985)
14. Regan, D. Low-contrast letter charts and sine wave grating tests in ophthalmological and neurological disorders. *Clinical Vision Sciences*, **2**, 235–250 (1988)
15. Rubin, M.L. The little point that isn't there. *Survey of Ophthalmology*, **17**, 52–53 (1972)
16. Harbin, T.S. Visual impairment by sunlight in posterior subcapsular cataracts. *Ophthalmic Surgery*, **4**, 34–36 (1973)
17. Paulsson, L.E. and Sjostrand, J. Contrast sensitivity in the presence of a glare light. *Investigative Ophthalmology and Visual Science*, **19**, 401–406 (1980)

18. Bernth-Petersen, P. Visual functioning in cataract patients. *Acta Ophthalmologica,* **59**, 198–205 (1981)

19. Nadler, M.P., Miller, D. and Nadler, D.J. *Glare and Contrast Sensitivity for Clinicians,* Springer-Verlag, New York (1990)

20. Holladay J.T., Prager T.C., Truillo T.C., Ruiz R.S. Brightness acuity test and outdoor visual acuity in cataract patients. *Journal of Cataract and Refractive Surgery,* **13**, 67–69 (1987)

21. Koch, D.D. Glare and contrast sensitivity testing in cataract patients. *Journal of Cataract and Refractive Surgery,* **15**, 158–164 (1989)

22. Elliott, D.B. and Hurst, M.A. Simple clinical techniques to evaluate visual function in patients with early cataract. *Optometry and Vision Science,* **67**, 822–825 (1990)

23. Wilkins, A.J., Della Sala, S., Somazzi, L. and Nimmo-Smith, I. Age-related norms for the Cambridge low contrast gratings, including details concerning their design and use. *Clinical Vision Sciences,* **2**, 201–212 (1988)

24. Pelli, D.G., Robson, J.G. and Wilkins, A.J. The design of a new letter chart for measuring contrast sensitivity. *Clinical Vision Sciences,* **2**, 187–199 (1988)

25. Kennedy, R.S. and Dunlap, W.P. Assessment of the Vistech contrast sensitivity test for repeated-measures applications. *Optometry and Vision Science,* **67**, 248–251 (1990)

26. Elliott, D.B. and Whitaker, D. Clinical contrast sensitivity chart evaluation. *Ophthalmic and Physiological Optics,* **12**, 275–280 (1992)

27. Bodis-Wollner, I. Visual acuity and contrast sensitivity in patients with cerebral lesions. *Science,* **178**, 769–771 (1972)

28. Regan, D., Silver, R. and Murray, T.J. Visual acuity and contrast sensitivity in multiple sclerosis – hidden visual loss: an auxiliary diagnostic test. *Brain,* **100**, 563–579 (1977)

29. van den Berg, T.J.T.P. Importance of pathological intraocular light scatter for visual disability. *Documenta Ophthalmologica,* **61**, 327–333 (1986)

30. Hess, R. and Woo, G. Vision through cataracts. *Investigative Ophthalmology and Visual Science,* **17**, 428–435 (1978)

31. Elliott, D.B., Gilchrist, J., Whitaker, D. Contrast sensitivity and glare sensitivity changes with three types of cataract morphology: are these techniques necessary in a clinical evaluation of cataract? *Ophthalmic and Physiological Optics,* **9**, 25–30 (1989)

32. Pardhan, S. and Gilchrist, J. The importance of measuring binocular contrast sensitivity in cataract. *Eye,* **5**, 31–35 (1991)

33. Elliott, D.B. How useful is the Vistech MCT8000 for contrast sensitivity and glare testing? *Canadian Journal of Optometry,* **54**, 194–198 (1993)

34. Ross, J.E., Bron, A.J. and Clarke, D.D. Contrast sensitivity and visual disability in chronic simple glaucoma. *British Journal of Ophthalmology,* **68**, 821–827 (1984)

35. Lennerstrand, G. and Ahlstrom, C.O. Contrast sensitivity in macular degeneration and the relation to subjective visual impairment. *Acta Ophthalmologica,* **67**, 225–233 (1989)

36. Elliott, D.B., Hurst, M.A. and Weatherill, J. Comparing clinical tests of visual function in cataract with the patient's perceived visual disability. *Eye,* **4**, 712–717 (1990)

37. van den Berg, T.J.T.P. On the relation between glare and stray light. *Documenta Ophthalmologica,* **78**, 177–181 (1991)

38. Elliott, D.B. and Bullimore, M.A. Assessing the reliability, discriminative ability and validity of disability glare tests. *Investigative Ophthalmology and Visual Science,* **34**, 108–119 (1993)

39. Ginsburg, A.P. A new contrast sensitivity vision test chart. *American Journal of Optometry and Physiological Optics,* **61**, 403–407 (1984)

40. Koch, D.D. and Liu, J.F. Survey of the clinical use of glare and contrast sensitivity testing. *Journal of Cataract and Refractive Surgery,* **16**, 707–711 (1990)

41. Rubin, G.S. Reliability and sensitivity of clinical contrast sensitivity tests. *Clinical Vision Sciences,* **2**, 169–177 (1988)

42. Brown, B. and Lovie-Kitchen, J.E. High and low contrast acuity and clinical contrast sensitivity tested in a normal population. *Optometry and Vision Science,* **66**, 467–473 (1989)

43. Bradley, A., Hook, J. and Haeseker, J. A comparison of clinical acuity and contrast sensitivity charts: effect of uncorrected myopia. *Ophthalmic and Physiological Optics,* **11**, 218–226 (1991)

44. Reeves, B.C., Wood, J.M. and Hill, A.R. Vistech VCTS 6500 charts: Within- and between-session reliability. *Optometry and Vision Science,* **68**, 728–737 (1991)

45. Elliott, D.B., Whitaker, D. and Bonette, L. Differences in the legibility of letters at contrast threshold using the Pelli–Robson chart. *Ophthalmic and Physiological Optics,* **10**, 323–326 (1990).

46. Elliott, D.B., Bullimore, M.A. and Bailey, I.L. Improving the reliability of the Pelli–Robson contrast sensitivity test. *Clinical Vision Sciences,* **6**, 471–475 (1991).

47. Bailey, I.L. Simplifying contrast sensitivity testing. *American Journal of Optometry and Physiological Optics,* **59**, 12P (1982)

48. Regan, D. The Charles F. Prentice Award Lecture 1990: Specific tests and specific blindnesses: Keys, locks, and parallel processing. *Optometry and Vision Science,* **68**, 489–512 (1991)

49. Adamsons, I., Rubin, G.S., Vitale, S., Taylor, H.R. and Stark, W.J. The effect of early cataracts on glare and contrast sensitivity: A pilot study. *Archives of Ophthalmology,* **110**, 1081–1086 (1992)

50. Rubin, G. *et al.* American Academy of Ophthalmology report: Contrast sensitivity and glare testing in the evaluation of anterior segment disease. *Ophthalmology,* **97**, 1233–1237 (1990)

51. Patorgis, C.J. Glare testing. In *Clinical Procedures in Optometry* (eds. J.B. Eskridge, J.F. Amos and J.D. Bartlett), J.B. Lippincott and Co., Philadelphia, pp. 487–492 (1991)

52. Miller, D., Jernigan, M.E., Molnar, S., Wolf, E. and Newman, J. Laboratory evaluation of a clinical glare tester. *Archives of Ophthalmology*, **87**, 324–332 (1972)

53. Bailey, I.L. and Bullimore, M.A. A new test for the evaluation of disability glare. *Optometry and Vision Science*, **68**, 911–917 (1991).

54. Elliott, D.B., Hurst, M.A. and Weatherill, J. Comparing clinical tests of visual loss in cataract patients using a quantification of forward light scatter. *Eye*, **5**, 601–606 (1991)

55. Tunnacliffe, A. Is routine contrast sensitivity measurement clinically useful? *Optician*, **201** (5302), 21–22 (1991).

56. Pardhan, S. and Elliott, D.B. Clinical measurements of binocular summation and inhibition in patients with cataract. *Clinical Vision Sciences*, **6**, 355–359 (1991)

57. Flammer, J. and Bebie, H. Lens opacity meter: A new instrument to quantify lens opacity. *Ophthalmologica*, **195**, 69–72 (1987)

58. Elliott, D.B. and Hurst, M.A. Assessing the progress of cataract. A clinical evaluation of the Opacity Lensmeter 701. *Optometry and Vision Science*, **66**, 257–263 (1989)

59. de Waard, P.W.T., IJspeert, J.K., van den Berg, T.J.T.P. and de Jong, P.T.V.M. Intraocular light scattering in age-related cataracts. *Investigative Ophthalmology and Visual Science*, **33**, 618–625 (1992)

60. Sparrow, J.M., Bron, A.J., Brown, N.A.P., Ayliffe, W. and Hill, A.R. The Oxford clinical cataract classification and grading system. *International Ophthalmology*, **9**, 207–225 (1986)

61. Chylack, L.T., Wolfe, J.K., Singer, D., Leske, M.C., Bullimore, M.A., Bailey, I.L., Wu, S.Y. and the LSC study group. The Lens Opacities Classification System, Version III (LOCS III). *Investigative Ophthalmology and Visual Science* (Supplement), **33**, 1096 (1992)

62. Taylor, H. and West, S.K. A simple system for the grading of lens opacities. *Lens Research*, **5**, 175–181 (1988)

63. Fincham, E.F. Photographic recording of opacities of the ocular media. *British Journal of Ophthalmology*, **39**, 85–89 (1955)

64. Kawara, T. and Obazawa, H. A new method for retroillumination photography of cataractous lens opacities. *American Journal of Ophthalmology*, **90**, 186–189 (1980)

65. Mishima, S. The use of polarized light in the biomicroscopy of the eye. *Advances in Ophthalmology*, **10**, 1–31 (1960)

66. Cope, W.T., Wolbarscht, M.L. and Yamanashi, B.S. The corneal polarisation cross. *Journal of the Optical Society of America (A)*, **68**, 1139–1140 (1978)

67. Bron, A.J. and Brown, N.A.P. Perinuclear lens retrodots: a role for ascorbate in cataractogenesis. *British Journal of Ophthalmology*, **71**, 86–95 (1987)

68. Widakowich, J. Cholesteric liquid crystals in the human cataractous lens observable with polarized light. *Acta Ophthalmologica*, **60**, 835–837 (1982)

69. Brown, N.A.P., Bron, A.J., Ayliffe, W., Sparrow, J. and Hill, A.R. The objective assessment of cataract. *Eye*, **1**, 234–246 (1987)

70. Niesel, P. Spaltlampenphotographie mit der Haag-Streit spaltlampe 900. *Ophthalmologica*, **151**, 489–504 (1966)

71. Brown, N. An advanced slit-image camera. *British Journal of Ophthalmology*, **56**, 624–631 (1972)

72. Dragomirescu, V., Hockwin, O., Weigelin, E. and Koch, H.R. The Scheimpflug photography of the anterior eye segment. Its application in cataract evaluation. In *Ageing of the Lens* (edited by F. Regnault, O. Hockwin and Y. Courtois), Elsevier, Oxford, pp. 301–306 (1980)

73. Datiles, M.B., Edwards, P.A., Trus, B.L. and Green, S.B. In vivo studies on cataracts using the Scheimpflug slit-image camera. *Investigative Ophthalmology and Visual Science*, **28**, 1707–1710 (1987)

74. Gilchrist, J. Computer processing of ocular photographs – A review. *Ophthalmic and Physiological Optics*, **7**, 379–386 (1987)

75. Sparrow, J.M., Brown, N.A.P., Shun-Shin, G.A. and Bron, A.J. The Oxford modular cataract image analysis system. *Eye*, **4**, 638–648 (1990)

76. Brubaker, R.F., Maurice, D.M. and McLaren, J.W. Fluorometry of the Anterior Segment. In *Non-invasive Diagnostic Techniques in Ophthalmology* (edited by B.R. Masters), Springer-Verlag, New York, pp. 248–280 (1990)

77. Zuclich, J.A., Glickman, R.D. and Menendez, A.R. In situ measurements of lens fluorescence and its interference with visual function. *Investigative Ophthalmology and Visual Science*, **33**, 410–415 (1992)

78. Zigman, S. Light filters to improve vision. *Optometry and Vision Science*, **69**, 325–328 (1992)

Assessment of retinal and neural function behind a cataract

Mark A. Hurst, William A. Douthwaite and David B. Elliott

6.1 Introduction

There are many instances when it is desirable to have some form of appraisal of the status of the visual pathway behind a cataract.

6.1.1 To provide additional information which can be used to aid diagnosis and management of visual loss

Most eye care professionals are familiar with the dilemma which confronts them when cataract seems to be the appropriate diagnosis but its degree does not seem to justify the measured visual loss. Similar predicaments impede diagnosis when cataract and one or more concurrent diseases are detected. This is especially so when a clear view of the macula is impossible.

In the Cardiff University-based low-vision clinic, where the commonest cause of low vision is age-related maculopathy, it was noted that cataract stands out as the most frequently found secondary condition contributing to the cause of low vision [1]. It is therefore likely that some of these patients could be helped by cataract extraction. A surgeon may be more confident of postsurgical improvement in this type of patient if the differential visual loss is known.

These dilemmas can usually be clarified by an assessment of the retinal and neural function behind the cataract. The results from this can then be used to aid correct diagnosis and management of the patient.

6.1.2 In anticataract drug trials or other longitudinal studies of cataract progression

As the cataract of a patient progresses, then a reduction in visual function usually takes place. Most methods of following cataract longitudinally give measures of visual function which can be influenced not only by cataract but also by a deterioration in retinal and/or neural function. It is therefore necessary that techniques that are capable of assessing retinal/neural function are included in the protocols of such studies. If this is the case, any change in visual function can then be isolated as being caused by a change in the status of the cataract, rather than by the possibility of a concurrent change in retinal/neural function.

6.1.3 To reduce the possibility of litigation as a result of disappointing postsurgical results of cataract extraction

Although at present this problem is more applicable to ophthalmic practice in the USA, there is no doubt that, in the future, the incidence of litigation will increase in the UK. The reasons for this are many, not least of which is the resounding success that the technique of intraocular lens implantation has achieved in the last 5–10 years. This success has, in turn, brought increased expectations from the patient awaiting cataract surgery. Many patients are now anticipating surgery at an earlier stage of visual impairment. As a consequence, the improvement in visual performance measured after the operation is not as striking as when typical pre operative acuities were 6/36. There is also increasing demand for 'second eye' surgery, which gives the obvious opportunity of comparing vision between the two eyes.

Some 22% of medicolegal claims in the USA are made with respect to cataract surgery, with the majority of these being related to intraocular lens implantation [2]. Indeed, there have been several instances when dissatisfied patients have won legal cases against ophthalmologists whose surgery was considered to be unjustified even when fully informed consent had been given.

It can be seen then that, where doubt arises with regard to the risk/benefit ratio of cataract surgery, some form of retinal/neural assessment giving information concerning the integrity of the visual pathway behind the cataract can help to justify the need for surgery.

6.2 Techniques

The problems outlined above are not all of recent origin; indeed several specialized methods have been developed over many years to improve the preoperative assessment of patients with cataract. Their clinical use is primarily when the routine tests of macular integrity, such as ophthalmoscopy, prove to be inconclusive. These methods can broadly be defined as belonging to the following categories.

6.2.1 Techniques that generally give only gross and rudimentary information about the integrity of the retina

The main advantage is that they can easily be carried out in the consulting room. Examples of these include the light projection test, two-light test, colour perception tests, various pinhole tests, Comberg's method, Maddox rod test and the trans-illuminated Amsler test. In locations where ophthalmic facilities are readily available, some of these tests have become largely redundant. The reason for this is because most patients now seek consultation well before the cataract has progressed to a stage that would justify carrying out tests of this gross nature. None-the-less, they can be of value where situations do not allow the use of more specialized equipment.

6.2.2 Entoptic phenomena

Demonstration of entoptic phenomena, such as Purkinje's vascular images and the blue-field entoptic phenomenon, has been said to give a subjective indication of normal retinal function.

6.2.3 Interference fringe techniques and the Potential Acuity Meter

These give precise subjective information in ways which attempt to be comparable with, and therefore predictors of, postoperative visual acuity (VA). Examples are the Rodenstock retinometer, the Lotmar Visometer and the Potential Acuity Meter (PAM).

6.2.4 Hyperacuity techniques

These give measurements which are independent of optical image degradation. Examples are vernier acuity and displacement thresholds.

6.2.5 Electrophysiology

These techniques give more objective information via electrical signals. Examples are the electroretinogram (ERG) and the visually evoked response/potential (VER/P). There are other electrophysiological techniques used in the clinical situation such as the electro-oculogram (EOG) and the electrically evoked response (EEG) but at the moment the ERG and the VER appear to be the most useful in terms of retinal/neural assessment behind cataract.

6.2.6 Ultrasound

Sound waves are used to determine the position of the components which make up the posterior layers of the eye. Ultrasound will indicate the presence of retinal detachment or vitreous haemorrhage for example.

6.3 Rudimentary clinical techniques

6.3.1 Projection test

Here the patient is asked to accurately demonstrate the location of a small light source by pointing towards it when it is held by the examiner in all four quadrants of the visual field. Unfortunately, dense cataracts interfere with accurate localization of point light sources, by scattering light on to the peripheral retina which would otherwise fall on the macular area. This limits the value of this test. However, the light source can also be used in an alternating manner to test for afferent pupil defects.

6.3.2 The swinging penlight test

The technique is to examine the patient in a darkened room. The light is shone into the good eye for 4 s and then quickly shifted to the other eye. If an afferent defect is present, both pupils will dilate. This is because the pupil response of the bad eye is being influenced, not only by its poor direct light response, but additionally by the consensual reflex of the now dilating good eye. Although this test works even with the densest cataracts, it is limited by the fact that the reflex is mediated not only by macular cones but also by those at the periphery of the retina.

6.3.3 Two-light test

The task here is simply to determine the minimum separation of two penlights that causes them to be seen as separate entities. This is, of course, a rough resolution test. The results can, however, be misleading when the possible angle of resolution in the presence of cataract is larger than the visual field permits. Thus, patients with reduced visual fields will have their standard of projection limited by visual field constraints rather than by the limits of resolution of the remaining intact field. Again, because of this, its value is limited. Although there are no apparent guidelines for the interpretation of the results, reasonable criteria were adopted by Sinclair *et al.* [3] who considered the response to be favourable if:

(a) The separation was $\leqslant 12.5$ cm for VAs of hand movements or light perception.
(b) The separation was $\leqslant 7.5$ cm for VAs of counting fingers to 6/60.
(c) The separation was $\leqslant 5$ cm for VAs better than 6/60.

6.3.4 Colour perception test

The technique here is to use perception of red, blue and green colours as an indicator of cone function. An appropriate filter from the trial case is held in front of the eye and a pen torch is shone through each filter into the patient's eye. Since many cones are outside the foveal area, this test is not a good indicator of macular function. The results are also influenced by the increased absorption of blue light, caused by the increased brunescence of nuclear cataract. This may account for its poor performance when used to predict macular function, giving, in one study, an 81% false negative rate [4].

6.3.5 Pinhole test

A black disc, perforated with 3 pinholes, approximately 1 mm in diameter and back-illuminated by a pen torch, is used in this test. The patient is required to count the holes and recount the pattern in which they are arranged. Alternatively, the multiple pinholes can be used by the patient to find the best view of the surroundings in a similar way to the use of a normal pinhole.

6.3.6 Comberg's method [5]

This technique, described by Goldmann [6], makes use of two bright light sources, such as a pair of identical pen torches or ophthalmoscopes, to indirectly test retinal function. One torch is placed before the right eye, the other before the left. Both light sources are brought forward towards the eye until the patient judges the illumination from both lights to be the same. If retinal function is equivalent in each eye, then the distance of the light sources from the eyes will also be equal. The test is obviously of most use in the presence of a uniocular cataract and a normal fellow eye.

6.3.7 Maddox rod test

Again, most useful in the case of uniocular cataract, a Maddox rod is placed in front of the cataractous eye and the patient asked to inspect the continuity of the red line created by the rod. The line should appear to be straight with no distortion or break.

6.3.8 Trans-illuminated Amsler test

This modified Amsler test was first described by Miller *et al.* [7]. Its 21 horizontal lines and 21 vertical lines are formed by a series of 1 mm holes (separated by 5 mm) drilled in a black board to fashion a grid measuring 10 cm by 10 cm. A 4 mm fixation hole is also drilled in the centre of the grid. The plastic board is mounted on a light box of the same size and the holes of the grid are therefore illuminated from behind by 2 × 44 cm neon tubes (15 W). Normal macular function is inferred if all the lines of dots appear straight, while abnormality is indicated if metamorphopsia or scotomas are reported. These criteria were adopted by Bernth-Peterson [4] when carrying out a pre- and post-operative comparison between this modified test and the colour perception test for macular function. He found that it was able to identify diseased maculae with 68% probability and normal maculae with a probability of 90%. Some 27% of his patients were unable to see the grid.

6.4 Tests to demonstrate entoptic phenomena

Entoptic phenomena are described as visual perceptions of normal or abnormal structures seen only under special conditions of illumination.

6.4.1 Self-ophthalmoscopy using Purkinje's vessel shadows

When a powerful trans-illuminating light is used against the sclera (thereby bypassing the lens), a shadow of the retinal vasculature falls on the receptors. This shadow is projected forward into space. Most patients are capable of appreciating these shadows, and, by subjective inspection of the pattern, are able to give information about the integrity of the retina. The technique, which is described by Goldmann [6], is to move the illuminating light back and forth in a vertical direction about 7 mm from the limbus, whereupon, Goldmann [6] claims, 80% of normal patients will appreciate the shadows. If the light is moved as described above in a vertical manner, then not only are vessel shadows seen but also a granular appearance of the foveal region is reported (this appearance is not seen if the light is moved horizontally). Goldmann [6] again claims that, if the appearance of this granular effect is used as a predictor of post-operative acuity, a positive response to this granular effect will give an expected post-operative VA of 6/12 to 6/6.

6.4.2 Blue field entoptic test

This phenomenon was first described over 200 years ago but was proposed as a clinical test of macular function by Scheerer [8]. It was noticed that, when a blue sky was viewed, numerous flying bright dots could be seen moving in a sinuous manner and usually in a series of accelerations and decelerations. The bright dots are now attributed to leucocytes flowing in the parafoveal capillaries [9]. The mechanism of their perception is said to be as follows. Haemoglobin in erythrocytes absorbs all the available blue light and therefore no stimulation of the retinal receptors occurs when blue light impinges on these cells. Leucocytes, however, contain no haemoglobin and therefore transmit blue light, which is then available to evoke the visual sensation, which manifests itself as the flying corpuscle effect. The series of accelerations and decelerations is synchronized with the cardiac cycle.

The situation in which these images can be seen has since been refined, whereupon it is now optimally demonstrated by viewing against a background illuminated by a blue light (430 nm) produced by a 500 W tungsten bulb. A commercially made instrument, the blue-field entoptoscope BFE 100 (Medical Instrument Research Associates; see Figure 6.1), is also available. The BFE 100 is used in a darkened

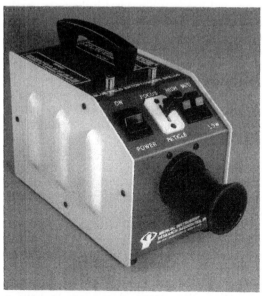

Figure 6.1 The blue-field entoptoscope BFE100 (Medical Instrument Research Associates).

room and the patient (usually with pupils dilated) looks down the eyepiece of the instrument to observe a 20° uniform blue field which is split into four quadrants by a black graticule. Refractive status is not important. The patient's first task is to notice the flying corpuscles. He or she is then asked to describe approximately how many there are in the field of vision, whether any quadrants have less than others, whether the sinuous movements are appreciated and, finally, if possible, whether the speed of movement is different between the two eyes.

Numerous studies have evaluated this technique [10–13] and have highlighted its advantages and disadvantages.

Certainly it is relatively easy under optimal conditions to see the flying corpuscles. Potter and Norden [10] reported that 99% of their normal patients were able to perceive them. Judgements regarding their position and quantity (at least 15 are suggested as being normal [3], although up to 30 may be seen) were seemingly more difficult to make, with 19.19% of normals seeing different numbers of corpuscles in at least one quadrant [10]. Since these discrepancies seemed to occur when more elderly patients were tested, it was inferred that these could be attributed to abnormalities in the parafoveal circulation, which were undetectable by fundoscopy [10]. Patients with cataract have been found to have even more difficulty [3]. Skalka [12] reported that the blue-field entoptoscopy test becomes a progressively more unreliable indicator of postoperative VA as cataract density increases, presumably because lens opacities reduce the retinal illumination. For those investigators able to modify their self-designed equipment merely by increasing the wattage of the light source, spectacular improvements in the numbers of cataract patients who could appreciate the corpuscles were obtained [3].

The quantity and position of the corpuscles is considered to be of importance but it has also been proposed that other observations could be made regarding their nature, which may have diagnostic implications [11].

Normal corpuscular movement is considered pulsatory, but Loebl and Riva [11] observed that some normal subjects (mainly those over 60 years of age), along with some with posterior pole disease, report uniform motion. The type of motion, they argue, does seem to have a relationship to the existence of retinal or systemic vascular disease, but this is not absolute. In the same study, other manifestations of the nature of the corpuscular flow in retinal disease were also noted, including an extension of scotomata found in the corpuscular field compared to that found with a 1/1000 white target. Slower comparative speeds of corpuscular movement in a diseased eye compared with that of a normal eye were considered to be of significance in relation to reduced blood flow.

Investigators assessing the efficacy of the technique of blue-field entoptoscopy in predicting the outcome of cataract surgery have assessed its merits by the number of false positives and false negatives produced during testing. In this regard, false negatives are patient responses that would indicate a properly functioning macula but that is subsequently shown to be unhealthy. Conversely, false positive responses indicate a poorly functioning macula that is in fact healthy.

Sinclair *et al.* [3] found that 94% of patients with normal maculae were identified correctly by the blue-field entoptic test (6% false positives). Of patients who were already diagnosed as having macular disease, poorly functioning maculae were identified in 90% of cases (10% false negatives). In a study involving patients who all had a variety of retinal pathology, similar numbers of false negatives (6%) were found [11]. These results seem to indicate that this technique does have some value in the prediction of postoperative retinal function.

Sinclair *et al.* [3] were fortunate enough to be able to increase the illumination of their blue-field equipment. Those who relied on the commercially available instrument in pre- and post-operative studies, such as Murphy [13], reported many problems. In particular, 45% of his patients with VAs of less than or equal to 6/30 before the operation, but better than 6/12 after the operation, were unable to see any corpuscles at all and were therefore classed as false positive.

Interestingly, when he divided his patients according to cataract morphology, he found that most of the false positives accrued from those patients with nuclear cataracts. He argued that because of their diffuse nature, nuclear cataracts tended to attenuate the blue-field illumination more than was caused by the more discrete posterior subcapsular cataracts. It appears, however, that only cataract classification for morphology was carried out with no mention of grading for extent. Despite this, his argument seems feasible, especially since most of the false positives found before the operation, were able to see the corpuscles after the operation. Other findings of interest from this study were that five out of the seven non-cataractous patients with, in his judgement, the most impaired macular function managed to see the corpuscles before surgery. It is of note that four of these patients had that most insidious condition, the macular hole. McDonnell *et al.* [14] have noted that macular holes do not demonstrate a deficient perifoveal vascular supply when subjected to fluorescein angiography. This may account for this condition giving false negative results with the blue-field entoptoscopy test.

A final point is worthy of note. The fovea is itself avascular and therefore the flying corpuscles are seen outside the perceived foveal area. Thus, loss of the phenomenon can still be concordant with good VA.

All the above tests give purely yes/no type responses. Results are therefore qualitative in nature and the degree of macular function can only be inferred. The benefit of the following techniques is that they give a quantitative prediction of the postoperative visual performance that can be expected.

6.5 Interference fringe techniques and the Potential Acuity Meter

6.5.1 Interference fringes

The philosophy behind the use of interference fringes is as follows. Optically created interference fringes are projected through a clear part of the lens on to the retina, where they are seen as alternate light and dark bands. The narrowest separation between an adjacent light and dark band that can be perceived gives a direct measure of the resolving power of the retina and neural system of the eye, since the optics are said to be bypassed.

In practice, the interference fringes are produced in one of two ways:

(a) by setting two high-frequency gratings (approximately 200 lines per mm) in contact and at an angle to each other, to form Moiré fringes derived from an incandescent light source;

(b) by using a pair of coherent light sources (usually a split helium–neon laser beam) to form the interference pattern.

These two methods of assessing retinal acuity were first described by Goldmann and Lotmar [15] (Moiré fringes) in 1969 and Green [16] (coherent light) in 1970 but only differ in the source from which the fringes are derived, rather than in major design differences. Each method generates a pair of point light sources near the pupil, the separation of which determines the width, or spatial frequency, of the interference fringes. The quality of these fringes is largely independent of the eye's refractive status (up to ± 10.00 D [17]), although very high ametropia can greatly reduce the number of fringes presented on the retina [18]. These qualities apart, this method of driving a target through the media, thereby bypassing the optics of the eye, has theoretical attractions for assessing retinal and neural function behind a cataract. In particular, the point light sources in both cases require a separation of less than 1 mm and this means it is possible to direct the twin beams towards and through a clear area of a cataractous crystalline lens (pupil dilatation is a necessity). Even if one of the beams is attenuated, it still may be possible to achieve a good-quality diffraction pattern.

Examples of commercially available instruments are the Rodenstock Retinometer (helium–neon laser, 633 λ, see Figure 6.2) and the Haag–Streit Visometer (incandescent light source) both of which mount on a slit-lamp. These instruments are capable of producing point sources, the separation of which can be varied to increase or decrease the spatial frequency of the fringes. Fringe orientation can also be varied to give horizontal, vertical and two oblique (45° and 135°) orientations. An example of a fringe produced by the Rodenstock Retinometer is shown in Figure 6.3. In these instruments, the spatial frequencies of the fringes have been calibrated by the manufacturers to provide a Snellen equivalent, ranging from 2/60 to 6/6 (Retinometer) and 6/60 to 6/3 (Visometer). Fields of view of the fringes produced by the retinometer are 5.5° and a choice of 1.5°, 2.5° and 3.5° by the Visometer.

The task for the patient is to correctly call the orientation of the grating. It is best to start with a fringe of low spatial frequency (wide gaps between bands) to give the patient some idea of

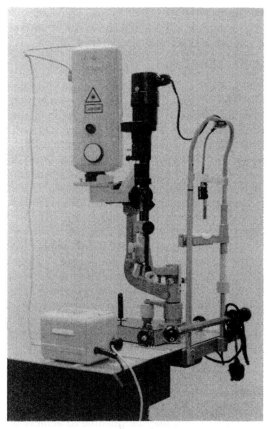

Figure 6.2 The Rodenstock Retinometer.

what is required. If the patient correctly calls two out of three different presentations, then the spatial frequency is increased (narrower bands) until one or less presentations are correctly called. The previous spatial frequency is then taken as the threshold of resolution and is recorded as a Snellen equivalent.

Not surprisingly, since each of these instruments are similar in operation, readings taken on the same subjects compare well with each other [19]; a correlation coefficient of 0.8, for example, has been quoted [17]. Unfortunately, in a study of non-cataractous patients, Geddes *et al.* [20] found a poor correlation between Snellen VAs and interferometric measurements.

The value of these instruments in predicting postoperative VA has been researched in depth, sometimes with contradictory conclusions. Halliday and Ross [17] found, in a pre- and postoperative study, that the Visometer gave a prediction of postoperative VA that was different from postoperative Snellen VA by ±25% in

45% of eyes that had only cataract. In eyes that had cataract and some other concurrent disease, the predictions were incorrect in 70% of cases. They concluded that the gratings penetrate the cataract but their quality is affected. The assumption that grating acuity is somehow equivalent to postoperative Snellen acuity was also questioned.

Faulkner [21,22] has studied the reasons for these poor predictions. In one of these investigations, he studied two groups of patients. One group had cataract but were otherwise quite normal, while the other group had cataract and macular disease. Although he found the rate of inaccurate predictions to be less than Halliday and Ross [17], he concluded that false positives and negatives were unacceptably high in several conditions.

False negatives were attributed to serous detachment of the sensory epithelium at the macula, cystoid macular oedema, glaucomatous field loss cutting through fixation, amblyopia, macular hole, pigmentary macular degeneration and early postoperative retinal detachment. It is argued that some of these diseases could be causing tilt of the retinal receptors. It is well known that tilted cells reduce Snellen VA, but as Faulkner [22] elegantly hypothesizes, it may be possible that they are still viable enough to produce a response to a grating.

False positive results were claimed to have accrued from testing patients with mature cataracts, vitreous haemorrhage and inadequate pupil dilatation.

Spurney *et al.* [23] disagreed with other investigators and concluded that overall the Visometer was a reliable predictor of postoperative VA. The majority of their patients had open-angle glaucoma, some with field loss not involving fixation, while others had dry age-related macular degeneration, i.e. mostly diseases not belonging to Faulkner's list. It is interesting to note that, when such patients were tested by other investigators [17,23,24], reports of inaccurate predictions usually followed. Moreover, if the results of every study were analysed overall, the correct prediction rate would appear to be excellent. This is not surprising since there were usually higher numbers of patients who had normal retinal function, compared with those who had concurrent disease, i.e. the predictive value of the test is open to influence from the prevalence of disease in the study population. If one considers the fact that the success rate (postoperative VAs better

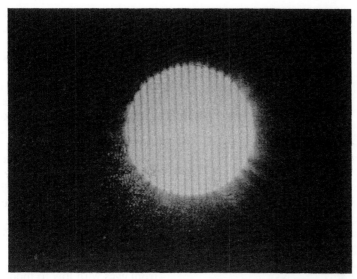

Figure 6.3 An example of an interference fringe produced by the Rodenstock retinometer.

than 6/12) of intraocular lens surgery was 89% in 1984 [25], equally favourable outcomes from surgery are possible to predict without the need for these instruments.

None-the-less, Enoch and his co-workers [18] felt that favourable interferometric results usually predicted good macular function. They did state, however, that their findings regarding poor results in the presence of cataract were indeed unreliable, since unfavourable results were not necessarily prognostic of poor postoperative VA. Commenting further on their results, they felt that preoperative interferometric measurements of 6/12 to 6/24 were of poor predictive value, since responses of this quality could be mediated by receptors which are distant from the fovea. Doubts regarding the use of the Visometer for quantitative predictions were also raised by Bernth-Peterson and Naeser [24] who found a poor correlation ($r = 0.07$) between the predicted result and the postoperative letter acuity.

6.5.2 The Potential Acuity Meter (PAM) (Mentor O&O)

This slit-lamp-mounted instrument (Figure 6.4), first described in 1981 [26], produces a single point light source of about 0.15 mm diameter in the plane of the pupil, which can be directed through clear areas of cataractous lenses in a similar way to the interferometers (see Section

6.5.1). This point light source generates an aerial image of a Snellen chart, with a field of view of 6°. This instrument must be focused (either by patient or examiner) to take account of patient ametropia. Ametropias of +15.00 DS to −10.00 DS are accounted for by an external knob located on the main body of the instrument. After pupil dilatation, the patient's task is to read the projected Snellen chart in the conventional way. Some adjustment of the ametropia setting, or position of the beam relative to the cataract, may be necessary during measurements in order to achieve the optimum result.

In the first pre- and post-operative clinical study using this instrument [27], it was found that the postoperative success (rated as a result of 6/12 or better) was predicted in 91% of cases. Limitations, it was said, were due to:

(a) dense cataracts when the beam was unable to penetrate the opaque lens;
(b) examiner inexperience
(c) the subjective nature of the test.

These limitations were seemingly reinforced by another study [28] which noted an inability to achieve results in 7.4% of patients because of the density of cataract. None-the-less, 92% of the remainder gave results within 1 Snellen line of the prediction. When compared with interferometers, results were less impressive [22,23]. The PAM consistently predicted poorer results

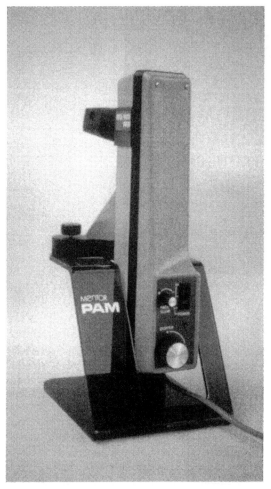

Figure 6.4 The potential acuity meter (PAM) (Mentor O&O).

do occur with both types of interferometer and the PAM. Their major drawback is their inability to reliably predict good postoperative acuity in cases of uncertain preoperative diagnoses. On the other hand, they may be of some use in quantitative rather than qualitative assessments.

(b)   Pupils must be maximally dilated.

(c)   Owing to the diffuse nature of even moderate nuclear lens opacities, it may not be possible to find an adequate window through which to direct the light beams.

(d)   Results may be unreliable in certain concurrent eye diseases, particularly when the condition could cause tilt of the retinal receptor cells. In these cases, false negative results are likely.

(e)   Results are most reliable when obtained from eyes with low to moderate degrees of cataract.

6.6 Hyperacuity measurements

The term hyperacuity [29] is used to describe a visual performance level above that achieved by measurements of maximum VA. If decisions regarding the spatial locations of two objects are to be made, rather than recognition of the objects as being separate entities (resolution), then the visual system is quite capable of making judgements about difference in position of less than 10 s of arc, hence the term hyperacuity.

Williams and his colleagues [30] were the first to argue strongly that some types of hyperacuity measurements could be used to assess vision behind media opacities and indeed could produce superior results to those obtained by interferometry, for example. The basis upon which this statement was made was primarily the strength of the resistance of 'two dot' vernier measurements to optical blur and also the fact that hyperacuity is highly dependent on retinal stimulus location, i.e. the lowest thresholds are achieved when the foveal area is stimulated [31].

There are several types of hyperacuity task; stereo acuity and vernier acuity are two examples.

(a)   Stereo acuity is the ability of a subject to detect differences in depth or distance of a pair or more of objects in space. Stereo

than were actually obtained after capsulotomy, for example. This was attributed to the fact that the PAM did not penetrate opaque media as well as interferometers. Particular problems again occurred when cataract was present along with the concurrent pathologies on Faulkner's [22] list.

The tendency of the PAM to give false positives had been noted earlier. Minkowski *et al.* [27] inferred that this tendency is a positive advantage since 'the PAM establishes a lower limit for VA which can be obtained by surgery'.

6.5.3 Summary

(a)   Care should be taken when interpreting results. False positives and false negatives acuity measurements fall in the same order of magnitude as other hyperacuities. They are, however, markedly affected by blur and therefore are unsuitable for the assessment of vision behind cataract.

(b)   Vernier acuity is the most well known of the hyperacuity tests. The target can consist of abutting vertical lines, two dots or vertical lines separated by a vertical gap. Here, the patient is asked to detect the misalignment of the lines or dots. The advantage of separating the lines vertically, as opposed to having an abutting line arrangement, is that the thresholds achieved are almost independent of target line length. Typical thresholds for this measurement are around 5 s of arc.

Conversely, the distance between dots in a 'two dot test' does influence measurements. Moreover, optimal thresholds are obtained at a specific separation for a particular standard of VA that an individual achieves. Several measurements therefore need to be made with different gaps between dots in order to optimize the measurement. A complementary measurement has also been proposed which can be allied to the results obtained from a 'two dot test', to produce a graph of thresholds varying with the degree of eccentricity. This has been termed 'gap perimetery' and involves measuring thresholds, not only when the subject is fixating centrally, but also when viewing eccentrically. The results from both these two measurements are compared with normative data and the quality of vision, attributed solely to the retinal and neural system, can then be predicted. Although this technique has been used clinically with some success [32], it is somewhat time consuming and ponderous.

Fortuitously, a more recently used hyperacuity test, that of displacement threshold measurement, is considerably quicker and more convenient to use than vernier acuities and gap perimetry. The task here is to determine the smallest change of position of an oscillating object which gives rise to the sensation of movement, when judged in relation to the position of two stationary reference bars. Thus, the oscillation is perceived as a displacement of the stimulus from the reference bars and not by its inherent movement. Here, thresholds of the order of 10 s of arc can be achieved, giving the test the properties of a hyperacuity test [33]. The

thresholds so obtained have also been shown to offer great resistance to image degradation by optical blur and mild cataracts [33,34]. Hence, a subject with a moderate degree of lens opacity would achieve the same thresholds both with and without the cataract. On the other hand, if the neural system behind the cataract is damaged, the hyperacuity threshold would be raised [32,35]. This has obvious application in predicting the visual outcome of cataract surgery and also for longitudinal studies on the progression of cataract.

A photograph of the equipment which can be used to measure the displacement threshold hyperacuity (DTH) is shown in Figure 6.5. The two outer reference bars are 5 min of arc wide, 45 min of arc high and are separated by a gap of 30 min of arc. Thresholds are derived from a yes/no staircase type of psychophysical procedure.

A similar arrangement has been used by Whitaker and Deady [35]. In this study they demonstrated that, not only are hyperacuity thresholds resistant to the image degradation caused by cataract, but also isolation of the amount of visual loss due to cataract from that caused by a damaged retinal/neural system is possible.

6.7 The electroretinogram (ERG) and the visually evoked response (VER)

There are basically two types of clinical electrophysiological techniques that could be considered for use as a means of assessing the integrity of the neural element of the visual system behind a cataract. These are the ERG and the VER. These two features are measured in a very similar manner. In both cases the patient is connected to the recording apparatus using:

(a)   An active electrode, which must be positioned close to the region of interest because this is the electrode which picks up the signal. In the ERG the active electrode is placed in contact with the anterior part of the eye. In the past, this was achieved by using a suitably modified contact lens but more recently the use of the Dawson–Trick–Litzkow (DTL) fibre has made ERG recording much easier and less traumatic for the patient [36,37]. DTL fibre is a low-mass electroconductive fibre which is

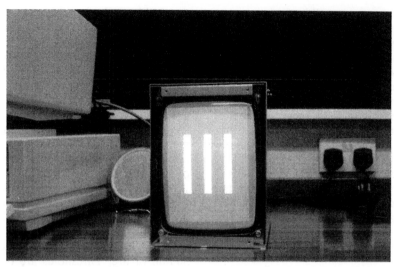

Figure 6.5 Monitor showing the central oscillating bar and the two flanking 'reference bars' used to measure displacement threshold hyperacuities. The two outer reference bars are 5 min of arc wide, 45 min of arc high and are separated by a gap of 30 min of arc.

simply laid across the lower lid margin of the patient, where it will pick up the ERG signal while at the same time inducing little or no discomfort. VER recording requires the active electrode to be attached to the scalp at the back of the head about 2 cm above the inion (the anatomical projection at the rear of the skull), if we wish to monitor macular activity.

(b) A reference electrode which completes the electrical circuit. This is placed in a position away from the region generating the signal so that it will pick up the general electrical activity. The use of a differential amplifier will then ensure that the signal which is amplified is that of the difference between the general electrical activity in the head and the electrical signal generated by the region involved in visual processing. The most common position recommended for the reference electrode is either the forehead or an ear lobe.

(c) A ground electrode. It is important that the patient and the recording equipment are electrically grounded in order to prevent artefact signals arising from electrical discharge between the patient and the equipment. The most common position for the ground electrode is on the forehead or an ear lobe.

In both the ERG and the VER, two basic types of stimulus can be used:

(a) A flashing diffuse stimulus.
(b) A patterned stimulus. This is usually a checkerboard pattern which either pattern reverses (the white and black checks interchange their positions at a predetermined rate) or cycles through a pattern onset/offset sequence.

The diffuse flash type target is ideal for cataract studies in that it can punch its way through the densest of cataracts. Indeed, it is possible to record responses through closed eyelids, if the discharge tube provides a sufficiently bright flash. This type of stimulation could be described as hitting the visual system with a sledge hammer. The resulting recordings, however, indicate the visual system response to light but give little, if any indication of foveal performance or integrity.

The pattern stimulus can be used in VER recording to assess macular and foveal function. The VER response is dominated by the macular signal as a result of two factors. First, the active electrode is in close proximity to the region of the visual cortex which processes macular information. Second, there is a considerable cortical magnification of the macular area, i.e. the proportion of cortex processing macular information is considerably larger than the proportional area of the retina covered by the macula. The macula projects on to approximately 50% of the occipital cortex, and so the VER is primarily an objective test of macular function. The foveal response can be further highlighted by using a pattern reversal checkerboard with small checks reversing at a slow rate to encourage spatial, rather than temporal, processing of the visual signal. In these circumstances, the amplitude of the VER shows a significant correlation with Snellen visual acuity [38]. Figure 6.6 shows VER waves obtained when using the small check size described above where it can be seen that the eye with the good VA is producing much larger waves than the amblyopic fellow eye.

The ERG, on the other hand, is a response which is dominated by the rods for the following reasons:

(a) The number of rods in the retina is considerably greater than the number of cones.
(b) The active electrode is positioned on the anterior part of the eye close to the retinal periphery, which is colonized almost entirely by rods.

The macula, which encompasses a 5° retinal area, only contains 1.5% of the total number of cones. Also, it has been shown that a 10% decrease in the cone function will not surpass

the variability of the ERG. Thus, lesions confined to the macula will not be detected by ERG examination. The flash ERG is a measure of gross retinal function which reflects the integrity of the photoreceptors and the bipolar cell layer. The flash ERG does not reflect the activity of the ganglion cell layer. Thus, a patient with glaucoma or optic nerve disease will probably have a normal ERG. The fact that the response is a measure of gross retinal function means that local disease such as macular degeneration may result in a normal ERG, whereas a diffuse retinal disease such as retinitis pigmentosa will result in an abnormal ERG.

For both the ERG and the VER, the macular, or indeed the foveal, response can be highlighted by using a checkerboard pattern with checks so small that only the foveal region is capable of resolving them. This type of target produces a VER wave where the amplitude correlates with the VA but a very weak ERG wave which is difficult to extract from the background noise with present recording techniques.

The major drawback associated with pattern stimuli, as with any other type of visual target containing fine detail, is that, if it is to be used to assess the neural integrity of the visual system, then a clear image of the target must be formed on the retina. This image must not be degraded by the presence of cataract. Clearly, this is not going to happen in the typical case and so the

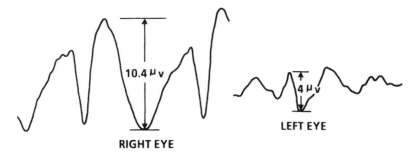

Miss G.M.K.

R.E. + 0.75 DS 6/5
L.E. + 0.75/ + 0.25 x 90 6/9
No strabismus
Fixation central and steady
V.E.R. to 5.5 min check at 6 reversals/sec

Figure 6.6 VER waves showing the amplitude attenuation produced by amblyopia. Right eye, +0.75 DS 6/5, left eye, +0.75 DS/+0.25 × 90 6/9. No strabismus. Fixation central and steady. VER to 5.5 min check at 6 reversals/s.

use of pattern stimuli to assess the neural response, independent of the cataract, will be of very limited value.

Returning, therefore, to the flash stimulus and considering the ERG, there appears to be a consensus that a normal preoperative ERG is a promising prognostic sign. The dominant feature of the ERG is a large positive wave called the b-wave. A diminished b-wave may precede a disappointing postoperative result. In fact the b-wave may be larger in the presence of cataract [39], particularly if a low stimulus intensity is employed [40]. It is suggested that this is due to the light-diffusing properties of the cataractous lens because it is known that a Ganzfeld diffuser produces an increase in amplitude with a shorter lasting b-wave in a normal eye. A Ganzfeld diffuser can easily be manufactured by cutting a hole in a table tennis ball and placing this 'diffusing sphere' over the eye, so that the whole of the retina is stimulated by diffuse light. Most cataracts, even those dense enough to preclude fundus observation, behave as intraocular Ganzfelds, and respectable ERG amplitudes may be expected in these circumstances.

Thompson and Harding [41] found that cataract had little effect on the amplitude and latency of the flash VER, provided that a high-intensity flash was used. They concluded that the flash VER can be used to predict the postoperative visual performance. It may be best, therefore, to record the flash ERG and VER, in order to maximize the potential information acquired. It is easy to record these two simultaneously.

Davis *et al.* [42] considered the presurgical prediction of postsurgical visual function in 112 cataract patients, using:

(a) the PAM;
(b) the laser interferometer;
(c) the blue-field entoptoscope;
(d) the bright-flash VER.

They performed a discriminant analysis to determine which test/s proved to be the most effective at diagnosing the presence of other vision-related diseases. They concluded that the flash VER was the most useful method of discriminating between cataract patients with concurrent neural complications and those without.

The rod contribution to the ERG can be minimized by using a bright flickering stimulus. This approach takes advantage of the fact that the rod response time is slower than that of the cones. If the stimulus is flashing at a sufficiently rapid rate, then the rods will be unable to resolve the temporal fluctuations and the ERG recorded will be derived from the cone system. Thus, flicker ERGs are considered to reflect more of the macular response and consequently this approach is a useful addition to any examination which is attempting to predict VA.

Weinstein [43] used a flash stimulus running at 10 Hz and recorded the VER which produced a double peak wave. He examined 90 subjects with opacities of the media (52 of these were cataract) and found a 67% agreement between the VER prediction of normal/abnormal VA and the actual postoperative acuity. He claimed that the amplitude of the second wave was attenuated in the presence of reduced VA and that this type of VER serves as an objective test of the predicted VA through opacities of the ocular media, as well as through closed eyelids. Thus, the non-patterned flash may yield information of prognostic value in media opacity cases.

Flash VER using rates of 1, 10 and 20 Hz have been used by Sherman and Cohen [44] who appear to be in agreement with Weinstein [43] when interpreting the 10 Hz response. They note, however, that a normal VER to a bright flash does not guarantee normal foveal functioning or a potentially normal VA, although it does suggest a favourable prognosis. If a VER cannot be recorded to a repetitive bright flash, then the potential for significant postoperative acuity improvement is remote. Transcleral stimulation using an optical probe applied to the lower lid has been suggested by Rubin and Dawson [45].

Vrijland and Van Lith [46] used photopic ERG and VER recordings on 350 patients and attempted to predict the postoperative visual performance. They concluded that a reasonable relationship exists between the ERG and VER on the one hand and VA on the other. This despite the reservations described above when ERG is used for assessment of the macula and considering the fact that photopic VERs also fail to detect pure foveal abnormalities.

6.8 Ultrasonography

Ultrasound is a form of sound wave which has a frequency above that which is audible. When an electric voltage is applied to a quartz crystal, the crystal oscillates at a particular frequency (10–20 MHz in ocular work) to produce sound waves. This crystal, or transducer, can also be used to receive a signal, which is then displayed by computer or oscilloscope. In practice, transducers are incorporated into a probe which is placed in fluid contact with the eye. In medical diagnostic work the equipment is designed to produce a low output, thereby avoiding destructive damage. Unfortunately, this means that the signals are more difficult to detect.

Two principal types of ultrasonographic display are available, dependent on the type of transducer and circuitry used:

(a) A scan. This time–amplitude display shows echoes as rising peaks from a time base which are related to each acoustic boundary within the eye, where the height of the echo is proportional to the amount of reflection from the interfaces. Therefore, echoes return from both surfaces of the cornea and both surfaces of the crystalline lens. In the case of cataract, reflections within the lens may be observed (Figure 6.7). The vitreous/retina border also produces an echo, with multiple reflections thereafter. Distances are dependent on the time it takes for the ultrasound to return. Thus a knowledge of velocities in each medium is necessary. In the case of cataract it is better to assume a velocity of 1550 m/s over the whole eye than guess at an unknown velocity in a seriously altered crystalline lens.

(b) B scan. This intensity-modulated display gives an anatomical cross-section of the eye. A sector-scanning transducer is usual but some are driven in a circle on a wheel and others move back and forth. A spot of light represents each echo on the screen, which varies in intensity according to the amount of reflection. Weaker echoes can, of course, be amplified with the gain control so that, for example, a vitreous detachment or haemorrhage can be spotted (Figure 6.8).

Patients are asked to move the eye during a B scan, so that the degree of mobility of echoes can be judged. In late-stage diabetic retinopathy, a mature cataract may co-exist with proliferative glial tissue or retinal detachment or both. Both

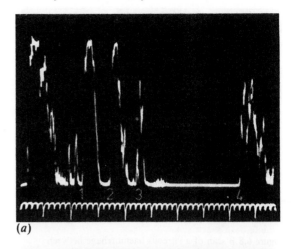

(a)

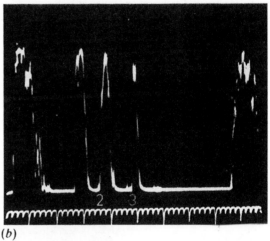

(b)

Figure 6.7(a) An axial A scan of a patient with advanced cataract. Echo 1 indicates the reflection from the cornea, 2 the anterior lens, 3 the posterior lens and 4 the retina. The spikes between 2 and 3 are produced by the cataract. (b) In a similar A scan of the fellow eye which possessed very little cataract there are no spikes between echoes 2 and 3.

of these are very reflective. The amount of mobility of these various echoes, after eye movement, can be a key diagnostic method for differentiation. A decision to carry out a vitrectomy and/or cataract surgery depends on the position of the retina (Figure 6.9).

Choroidal detachment with vitreous haemorrhage can occur after cataract surgery. The 'kissing effect' (Figure 6.10), where the echoes balloon towards each other, is a typical ultrasound display.

In general terms, A scan is more useful for precision of measurement and B scan is better

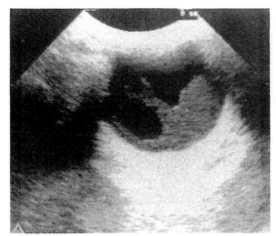

Figure 6.8 B scan of a vitreous haemorrhage between posterior vitreous detachment and retina at high amplification.

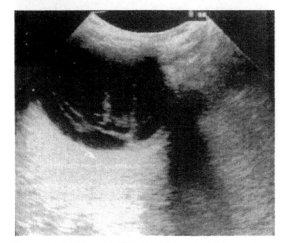

Figure 6.9 Proliferative diabetic retinopathy with traction on the retina.

slightly out of tune. Gilchrist and Pardhan [47] proposed that isolation of the neural and optical components of the human visual function might be achieved by measuring the contrast sensitivity of target images embedded in a background of visual noise. This measurement is called the contrast detection in noise (CDN).

The visual noise masks, or hides, the targets to be perceived. In general, adding visual noise will reduce the subjective sensitivity towards a target. As several levels of noise are used, the relationship between contrast sensitivity and noise may be determined. Gilchrist and Pardhan [47] and Kersten *et al.* [48] found discriminating changes of CDN in neurally based disease of the eye. Such changes were not observed in defects of the eye which were purely optical in origin.

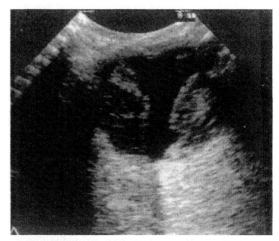

Figure 6.10 Choroidal detachment showing the kissing effect.

by far for assessment of pathology behind cataract. However, where tumours are present (Figure 6.11), a knowledge of the reflective qualities of the tumour with A scan can be very helpful in deciding on the type of tumour present.

6.9 Noise charts

Radio reception is degraded by interference (noise) in areas of poor reception. In a similar way, visual noise is said to mask the object of regard and hence reduce its visibility. The noise interferes with the view in a manner not unlike that of observing a television picture that is

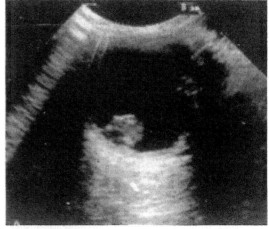

Figure 6.11 Malignant melanoma.

Two factors are of particular interest as far as visual noise is concerned:

(a) the amount of internal noise residing within the observer;
(b) the amount of external noise in the object of regard.

The effects of visual noise on contrast detection for example are shown in Figure 6.12. The *y*-axis represents the contrast threshold and a high value indicates low sensitivity, in the sense that the target must have a high contrast before it is perceived. The target has a single fixed spatial frequency.

The *x*-axis represents noise density which is linearly proportional to the square of the mean noise contrast. The appearance of the noise mask resembles a grainy background image which is superimposed on the target, so that the overall picture looks like a high-speed photographic print taken at low light levels. Thus, a high noise spectral density indicates that there is a large difference in the luminance (brightness) between the bright and dark parts of the noise mask and this will require a higher contrast in the target, if it is still to be perceived.

In Figure 6.12 contrast detection for a sine-wave grating is plotted against visual noise for three hypothetical observers. Thus, for all three subjects, the target contrast must be increased for it to be perceived when the mean noise contrast (noise density) is increased.

The *x* intercept represents the internal noise of the observer and this is called the equivalent noise. The perfect observer would show zero equivalent noise. The human observer never reaches this level. The internal noise in the human visual system can easily be observed by sitting in a totally dark room with closed eyes, whereupon the view does not look black but is seen to shimmer as a result of spontaneous firing of the receptors. The equivalent noise can be affected by both optical and neural changes within the visual system and so is of limited value when assessing the neural function behind a cataract. When compared with conventional contrast sensitivity measurement, however, it appears to hold promise as a more sensitive test for monitoring cataract development [49].

For the assessment of neural function behind a cataract, the gradient of the graph is the important parameter. The reciprocal of the gradient of the graph actually gives a measure of the neural efficiency of that particular subject

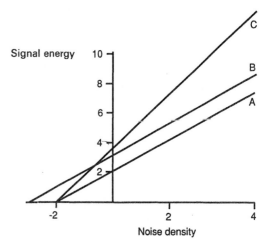

Figure 6.12 Effects of visual noise on contrast detection for three hypothetical observers. Line A is the response of a normal observer. Line B is the response of an observer with cataract and line C is the response of an observer with neural dysfunction. The *x* intercept is a measure of background noise of the visual system. The slope is a measure of visual processing efficiency.

and this is called the sampling efficiency. The perfect observer has a sampling efficiency of 1 or 100%.

If the sampling efficiency of the subject is poor, then the slope of the graph is steeper (subject C in Figure 6.12). This indeed has been shown to occur in patients with amblyopia [49] and diabetic retinopathy [50] for example.

In cataract (subject B in Figure 6.12), the type of slope obtained is similar to that of the normal observer (subject A), but in these cases there is usually a marked increase in the amount of internal noise (the *x* intercept on the graph). Thus, sampling efficiency is not affected by cataract but the equivalent noise is increased [47,48].

If a patient has a cataract and co-existing neural disease, then the slope will be steeper (reduced sampling efficiency) than if only a cataract was present. It is assumed that reduced sampling efficiency indicates the presence of a neural problem. However, only a limited number of neural conditions have been investigated to date. There is, therefore, the possibility that some neural defects may not affect sampling efficiency.

The problem of taking measurements such as those described above is their tedious nature. Gilchrist and Pardhan [47] and Beh [50] have developed a low-contrast letter test which can be used to assess both letter contrast sensitivity and neural efficiency quickly and easily. The current recommendation is to use two charts. The first chart consists of low-contrast targets with a zero noise level (Figure 6.13). This is similar to the Pelli–Robson chart (see Section 5.6.2). The second is a cognate chart in which is embedded a precalculated amount of added noise (Figure 6.14).

Both charts consist of nine lines of Landolt E letters arranged in groups of four (of the same contrast). The charts are viewed from a distance of 1 m, giving an equivalent size to a 60 m letter viewed at 6 m. The patient is simply asked to

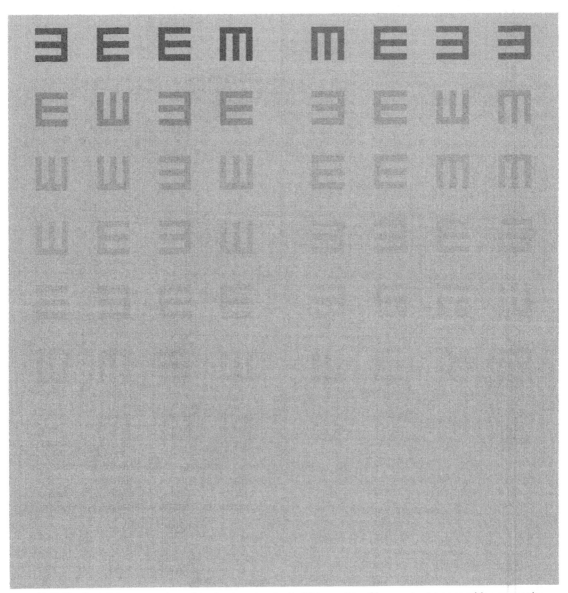

Figure 6.13 The first of the two contrast detection in noise charts. This consists of low-contrast targets with a zero noise level background.

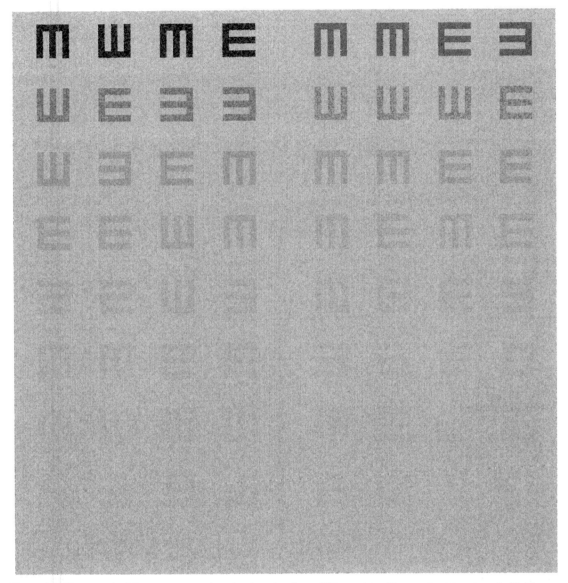

Figure 6.14 The second of the two contrast detection in noise charts. This consists of low-contrast targets embedded in background noise.

indicate the orientation of each E, starting with the letters of high contrast, until a threshold is reached with the letters of lower contrast. Similar precautions to those taken when using the Pelli–Robson chart are advised, such as allowing sufficient time to see letters near threshold.

Threshold results from both charts are recorded and the sampling efficiency and the equivalent noise of the patient can be determined by using a simple conversion table. Patients with normal neural function behind the cataract will show an increased equivalent noise (due to the cataract) with an unchanged sampling efficiency. A decrease in the sampling efficiency suggests a deterioration in the neural function behind the cataract.

6.10 Concluding remarks

For all the reasons quoted at the beginning of this chapter, research is continuing in this fascinating area of retinal and neural function assessment. New techniques which may have application in this field are continually being proposed and evaluated. Davis *et al.* [42], for example, have postulated that VERs obtained using a laser speckle stimulus may combine the advantages of both monochromatic laser interferometry and the flash VER. More recently, image processing has been utilized to restore the quality of captured fundal images of a cataractous eye [51], and the scanning laser ophthalmoscope will provide greater detail of the posterior part of the eye.

Some of the techniques described in this chapter have not yet found their way into established clinical practice. They remain in the domain of the clinical researcher and are, therefore, still being improved. Nevertheless, our description of these techniques must make it obvious to the reader that there is, as yet, no single test capable of providing an unequivocal answer to the question concerning the possibility of concurrent neural disease behind the cataract.

Acknowledgements

We wish to acknowledge the help of the late Dr John Storey, Ph.D., M.Sc., F.B.C.O., D.C.L.P., Principal Optometrist at the Manchester Royal Eye Hospital, UK, for his helpful comments on the text and the supply of the illustrations in the ultrasonography section of this chapter. We would also like to thank Butterworths for permission to use Figure 6.7 which has previously been published in the book *Optometry*.

References

1. Leat, S.J. and Rumney, N.J. The experience of a university-based low vision clinic. *Ophthalmic and Physiological Optics*, **10**, 8–15 (1990)
2. Bettman, J.W. Seven hundred medi-legal cases in Ophthalmology. *Ophthalmology*, **97**, 1379–1384 (1990)
3. Sinclair, S.H., Loebel, M. and Riva, C.T. Blue field entoptic test in patients with ocular trauma. *Archives of Ophthalmology*, **99**, 464–467 (1981)
4. Bernth-Peterson, P. Evaluation of the transilluminated Amsler grid for macula testing in cataract patients. *Acta Ophthalmologica*, **59**, 57–63 (1981)
5. Comberg, W. Lichtsinnprufung bei einseitiger Augenerkrankung mit Hilfe des Augenspiegels. *Vershandlungon der Deutschen für Ophthologie* **52**, 431 (1938)
6. Goldmann, H. Examination of the fundus of the cataractous eye. *American Journal of Ophthalmology*, **73**, 309–320 (1972)
7. Miller, D., Lanberts, D.W. and Perry, H.D. An illuminated grid for macular testing. *Archives of Ophthalmology*, **96**, 901–902 (1978)
8. Scheerer, R. Die entoptishe Sichtbarkeit der Blutbewegug im Auge und ihre klinishce Bedeutung. *Klinische Monatsblatter für Augenheilkunde*, **73**, 67–107 (1924)
9. Schmidt-Gross, U. Entoptishe Beurteilung der Leukocytenzahl. *Klinische Wochenschrift*, **32**, 817–819 (1954)
10. Potter, J.W. and Norden, L.C. Blue field entoptic test with normal patients. *Journal of the American Optometric Society*, **54**, 1075–1078 (1983)
11. Loebel, M.L. and Riva, C.E. Macular circulation and flying corpuscles phenomenon. *Transactions of the American Academy of Ophthalmology and Otoloryngology*, **85**, 911–917 (1978)
12. Skalka H.W. Blue field entoptoscopy and VER in preoperative cataract evaluation. *Ophthalmic Surgery*, **12**, 642–645 (1981)
13. Murphy, G.E. Limitations of blue field entoptoscopy in evaluating macular function. *Ophthalmic Surgery*, **4**, 1033–1036 (1983)
14. Mcdonnell, P.J., Fine, S.L. and Hillis, A. Clinical features of idiopathic macular cysts and holes. *American Journal of Ophthalmology*, **93**, 777–786 (1982)
15. Goldmann, H. and Lotmar, W. Beitrag zum porblem der bestimmung dr retinal sehscharfe bei katarakt. *Klinische Monatsblatter für Augenheilkunde*, **154**, 324–329 (1969)
16. Green, D.G. Testing the vision of cataract patients by means of laser generated interference fringes. *Science*, **168**, 1240–1242 (1970)
17. Halliday, B.L. and Ross, J.E. Comparison of 2 interferometers for predicting visual acuity in patients with cataract. *British Journal of Ophthalmology*, **67**, 273–277 (1983)
18. Enoch, J.M., Bedell, H.E. and Kaufman, H.E. Interferometric visual acuity testing in anterior segment disease. *Archives of Ophthalmology*, **97**, 1916–1919 (1979)
19. Lotmar, W. Apparatus for the measurement of retinal visual acuity by Moire fringes. *Investigative Ophthalmology and Visual Science*, **19**, 393–400 (1980)
20. Geddes, L.A, Patel, B.J. and Bradley, A. Comparison of Snellen and interferometer visual acuity in an ageing noncataractous population. *Optometry and Vision Science*, **67**, 361–365 (1990)
21. Faulkner, W. Laser interferometric prediction of postoperative visual acuity in patients with cataract. *American Journal of Ophthalmology*, **95**, 626–636 (1983)
22. Faulkner, W. Predicting acuities in capsulotomy

patients: Interferometers and potential acuity meter. *American Journal of the Intra-ocular Implant Society,* **9**, 434–437 (1983)

23. Spurney, R.C., Zaldivar, R., Belcher, C.D. and Simmons, R.J. Instruments for predicting visual acuity: A clinical comparison. *Archives of Ophthalmology* **104**, 196–200 (1986)

24. Bernth-Peterson, P. and Naeser, K. Clinical evaluation of the Lotmar Visometer for macular testing in cataract patients. *Acta Ophthalmologica (Kbh),* **60**, 525–532 (1982)

25. Southwick, P.C and Olson, R.J. Shearing posterior chamber intraocular lens implantation. *Journal of the American Intraocular Implant Society,* **10**, 318–323 (1984)

26. Minkowski, J.S. and Guyton, D.L. Potential Acuity Meter using a minute aerial pinhole aperture. *Ophthalmology,* **9** (Suppl), 95 (1981)

27. Minkowski, J.S., Palese, M. and Guyton, D.L. Potential Acuity Meter using a minute aerial pinhole aperture. *Ophthalmology,* **90**, 1360–1368 (1983)

28. Christenbury, J.D. and Mcpherson, S.D. Potential Acuity Meter for predicting post-operative visual acuity in cataract patients. *American Journal of Ophthalmology,* **99**, 365–366 (1985)

29. Westheimer G. Visual acuity and hyperacuity. *Investigative Ophthalmology and Visual Science,* **14**, 570–572 (1975)

30. Williams, R.A., Enoch, J.M. and Essock, E.A. The resistance of selected hyperacuity configurations to retinal image degradation. *Investigative Ophthalmology and Visual Science* **25**, 389–399 (1984)

31. Westheimer, G. The spatial grain of the perifoveal visual field. *Vision Research,* **22**, 157–162 (1982)

32. Enoch, J.M., Williams, R.A., Essock, E.A., and Fendick, M. Hyperacuity perimetry: Assessment of macular function through ocular opacities. *Archives of Ophthalmology,* **102**, 1164–1168 (1984)

33. Whitaker, D. and Buckingham, T. Oscillatory movement displacement thresholds: resistance to optical image degradation. *Ophthalmic and Physiological Optics,* **7**, 121–125 (1987)

34. Whitaker, D. and Elliott, D.B. Towards establishing a clinical displacement threshold technique to evaluate visual function behind cataract. *Clinical Vision Sciences,* **4**, 61–69 (1989)

35. Whitaker, D. and Deady, J. Prediction of visual function behind cataract using displacement threshold hyperacuity. *Ophthalmic and Physiological Optics,* **9**, 20–23 (1989)

36. Dawson, W.W., Trick, G.L. and Litzkow, C.A. Improved electrode for electroretinography. *Investigative Ophthalmology and Visual Science,* **18**, 988–991

(1979)

37. Thompson, D.A. and Drasdo, N. An improved method for using the DTL fibre in electroretinography. *Ophthalmic and Physiological Optics,* **7**, 315–319 (1987)

38. Douthwaite, W.A., Jenkins, T.C.A. and Taylor, A. J. Visual acuity prediction using the VER – temporal aspects. *American Journal of Optometry and Physiological Optics,* **64**, 888–896 (1987)

39. Mikawa, T. and Tamura, O. Relation between the electroretinogram and post operation vision in cataract. *Japanese Journal of Clinical Ophthalmology,* **24**, 43–46 (1970)

40. Burian, H.M. and Burns, C.A. A note on senile cataracts and the electroretinogram. *Documenta Ophthalmologica,* **20**, 141–149 (1966)

41. Thompson, C.R.S. and Harding, G.F.A. The visual evoked response in patients with cataracts. *Documenta Ophthalmologica (Proceedings)* **15**, 193 (1978)

42. Davis E.T., Sherman, J., Bass, S.J. and Schnider, C.M. Pre-surgical prediction of post-surgical visual function in cataract patients: Multivariate statistical analyses of test measures. *Clinical Vision Sciences,* **6**, 191–207 (1991)

43. Weinstein, W. W. Clinical aspects of the visually evoked potential. *Ophthalmic Surgery,* **9**, 56–65 (1978)

44. Sherman, J. and Cohen, J. Pre-surgical evaluation of the patient with cataract. *Southern Journal of Optometry,* **22**, 20–27 (1980)

45. Rubin, M. and Dawson, W. The transcleral VER: prediction of post-operative acuity. *Investigative Ophthalmology and Visual Science,* **17**, 71–74 (1978)

46. Vrijland, H.R. and Van Lith, G.H.M. The value of pre operative electro-ophthalmological examination before cataract extraction. *Documenta Ophthalmologica,* **55**, 153–156 (1983)

47. Gilchrist, J.M. and Pardhan, S. Contrast thresholds for gratings in noise: a new method for assessing visual function. *11th European Conference on Visual Perception,* Bristol (1988)

48. Kersten, D., Hess, R.F. and Plant, G.T. Assessing contrast sensitivity behind cloudy media. *Clinical Vision Sciences,* **2**, 143–158 (1988)

49. Pardhan, S., Gilchrist J. and Beh G.K. Contrast detection in noise. A new method for assessing visual function in cataract. *Optometry and Vision Science,* **70** (1993)

50. Beh, G.K. Clinical applications of contrast sensitivity in visual noise. Ph.D. thesis, University of Bradford (1992)

51. Pelli, E. and Pelli, T. Restoration of retinal images obtained through cataract. *Eye EEE Transactions on Medical Imaging,* **8**, 401–406 (1989)

The surgical management of age-related cataract

John R. Weatherill

7.1 Pre-operative assessment

7.1.1 General considerations

The development of the intraocular lens (IOL) implant, in conjunction with modern extracapsular surgery, has revolutionized the management of cataract. Today, one can offer cataract surgery to any patient whose opacities are interfering with their enjoyment of life. As already explained, Snellen acuity is not a reliable guide to the degree of handicap (see Section 4.3.4). In practice, the decision to operate depends on an assessment of the patient's needs, balanced against the risk of complications of surgery, which are infrequent but cannot be ignored.

Important general considerations are the patient's expectations and beliefs. Some people seem genuinely quite unconcerned by visual impairment that most would consider severely restricting, others are anxious to have the slightest defect corrected. In trying to gauge the patient's reaction to their disability, it should be remembered that many patients are frightened at the prospect of eye surgery and denial of symptoms may be used to avoid an operation. Folk memory is surprisingly long and many believe that cataracts cannot be removed until they are 'ripe' or fully mature and the patient is quite blind. Some believe that the operation is

painful and that both eyes have to be padded for several days following surgery. A less common but real fear is that the cataract is a form of 'growth' and irreversible changes will occur unless the operation is performed. It is important therefore to dispel the many myths that surround 'cataracts' before deciding on the best plan for any particular individual.

In order to advise patients on the likely benefit of an operation, the surgeon must have some knowledge of their way of life. Does the patient drive, particularly at night, use buses or need to be able to walk safely unaccompanied in busy traffic? Does the patient have particular recreations or hobbies which are becoming adversely affected by cataract? Many elderly patients find that their enjoyment of golf is spoilt by an inability to follow the ball's flight. Is viewing the television difficult and does the patient need to read teletext? Does the patient have dependants who rely on them to shop, read correspondence and check syringes and tablets? The assessment of a patient's near-vision requirements can be difficult because although everyone, if asked, would like to read newsprint fluently, in practice many patients read very little by choice rather than by inability to see.

In a reasonably healthy patient with no other ocular problem, there is no reason why any cataract should not be removed if it is interfering with their enjoyment of life. It is not uncommon to remove posterior subcapsular opacities from active patients when the Snellen acuity is better than 6/9.

7.1.1.1 When to refer

Ideally the patient with a cataract should be referred as soon as the opacity is causing symptoms. In practice, this may not be welcomed by the ophthalmologist because, in most parts of the UK, there is a long waiting time for out-patient referrals to be seen with an equally long waiting list for cataract surgery. If it can be ascertained whether a patient would, or would not, be willing to have an operation, then this may curtail a few unnecessary referrals. Far more commonly, we see patients who have relatively dense cataracts who are keen to have surgery as soon as possible. If these patients had been referred earlier, it would have been to their personal advantage, although earlier referrals lengthen surgical waiting lists.

The relatively low incidence of cataract surgery in the UK in contrast with the USA is probably due to under treatment in the former rather than over treatment in the latter. All health care professionals have a duty to give the best advice to their patients. If referral seems appropriate, this should be recommended, despite the fact that other claims on the public purse may be considered to have a higher priority than cataract surgery. There is never an easy answer to this dilemma but it is surely better to put patients forward for treatment, for which they might have to wait, rather than to deny them the prospect of improved vision on the grounds that resources, at the present time, are inadequate.

7.1.1.2 Old age

Old age is, of itself, no bar to cataract surgery, indeed the very old are frequently excellent candidates for surgery carried out under local anaesthesia. If the patient has a medical condition that can be cured, or at least improved, then this should be done. Surgery can be performed safely on all but the most seriously ill. Economists might argue that it is not worth operating on patients with a limited life expectancy but many of those affected take the opposite view, on the grounds that if one's days are numbered each day of sight is very precious.

7.1.1.3 Cataracts in children

Cataracts in children pose particular difficulties in management and, these days, are usually treated by paediatric ophthalmologists. Before the operation, one needs to know if the cataract is uni-ocular or binocular, whether it has been short or long standing and if there are any other ocular or systemic abnormalities. The main concern in these children is the possibility that amblyopia may be present or may be developing.

The infant's nucleus is very soft, and the whole lens can be aspirated relatively easily. As the posterior capsule opacifies quickly, many surgeons recommend removing the posterior capsule and anterior vitreous as part of the primary procedure. IOLs can be inserted into the infant's eye but this is not a routine method of correcting aphakia in an eye which is still developing. After surgery, the aim of treatment is to prevent amblyopia. These children need to be closely monitored to ensure that they do not develop intraocular inflammation leading to vitreous opacities.

7.1.2 Associated ocular conditions

Having elicited any previous history of ophthalmic problems and any family history of eye disease, which might be more of a concern to the patient than of relevance to their present condition, the surgeon examines the eyes in order to answer two questions:

(a) Are the cataracts the cause of the patient's symptoms?
(b) If so, are there any associated conditions that might prejudice the successful outcome of cataract extraction?

The assessment of the cataract has been discussed at length elsewhere in this book but, in summary, nuclear cataract progresses slowly and appears to cause surprisingly little handicap, and posterior subcapsular opacities advance more quickly and are troublesome at an early stage of development.

Associated ocular conditions affect the decision to operate in two ways. There are those that impair vision, such as corneal opacities and macular degeneration, and those that threaten vision, such as glaucoma and untreated adnexal infections.

It would be tedious and unnecessary to list all the possible ocular findings but some signs concerning the pupillary reactions and the iris are particularly important. No matter how dense the cataract, the pupils should show a brisk direct and indirect reaction to light. A relative afferent pupillary defect suggests posterior segment pathology and requires investigation. A fixed pupil may be the only sign of a long-forgotten iritis. Tiny notches in the sphincter of the iris suggest blunt trauma and possible retinal damage. Heterochromia may also be due to previous trauma and is also seen in Fuch's cyclitis, the 'commonest missed ophthalmic condition'. Segmental iris atrophy may be due to intermittent angle closure. Tiny flecks of exfoliative material warn of possible glaucoma, and retro-illumination will reveal albinism.

7.1.2.1 The only eye

In general, cataract surgery is safe but there are some rare complications which may destroy the sight completely and so, if a patient has only one eye, both patient and surgeon should be cautious. The time-honoured principle is not to risk surgery whilst the patient has some useful sight so that the operation is only performed when the patient has little to lose. This policy condemns some patients to years of poor sight, in many cases quite unnecessarily but there is no easy answer to the dilemma. Although one may advise a patient quite accurately, in the statistical sense, of the risks involved, one also has to take into account the perception of risk. This is a wide and fascinating subject. It appears that we are quite prepared to accept high risks if we believe we are in control of a situation, for example when driving or smoking, but we react with horror to much lower risks over which we have no control, such as ionizing radiation. The perception of surgical risks falls between these two extremes, and individual reactions to possible complications vary enormously. Similar problems arise when the patient has other ocular conditions affecting the sight of both eyes. Usually, the poorer eye is operated on first but not every patient appreciates this cautious approach, as the result of the first operation may be disappointing. In practice, we find that once a patient has experienced the first operation, they are usually surprised at how little pain, discomfort or morbidity is experienced and readily agree to the second procedure.

7.1.2.2 Age-related macular degeneration

It is worth emphasizing that it is almost impossible to accurately predict visual acuity (VA) from the fundus appearance. The most treacherous condition is the 'foveal hole', a degeneration confined to the fovea, which causes severe loss of vision, and which can be extremely difficult to detect when the view is obscured by lens opacities. The use of the 78 D or 90 D lens is the best way to find this elusive lesion. Occasionally, dense cataracts are removed from patients with known macular degeneration so as to improve peripheral vision but the end result is often disappointment for the patient.

7.1.2.3 Myopia

Myopia is a condition that affects many structures of the eye and myopic patients may have pre-existing retinal problems and glaucoma as well as postoperative complications such as retinal detachment. The relationship of retinal detachment to cataract surgery is twofold. Some, usually myopic, patients develop detachment after uncomplicated extracapsular cataract extraction and in these patients the detachment and cataract are considered to be a reflection of the somewhat degenerate nature of the myopic eye. If, however, there has been rupture of the posterior capsule, or in addition, vitreous loss, then there is an increased incidence of retinal detachment. In other words, most surgeons would agree that an uncomplicated extracapsular extraction is not of itself associated with retinal detachment. Although very few surgeons would recommend clear lens extraction and IOL implantation to correct high myopia, there is no doubt that the restoration of emmetropia to myopic patients with cataracts is of enormous optical benefit and these patients in particular are usually very keen to have bilateral surgery.

7.1.2.4 Glaucoma

Glaucomas and cataracts are linked in many ways. Cataract may cause glaucoma and indirectly glaucoma may cause cataract. More usually these two common conditions occur in the same patient by chance. The two most important questions to be asked in this context are:

(a) Has the glaucoma destroyed so much visual field that cataract extraction would be useless or even dangerous?

It is known that intraocular procedures in patients with severely restricted fields of vision can lead to complete loss of sight. A relative afferent pupillary defect would be an indication of extensive glaucomatous damage.

(b) Is the glaucoma well controlled or is a trabeculectomy necessary?

The aims of the two operations are diametrically opposed in that the trabeculectomy forms a continuously draining fistula but in cataract surgery we aim for a watertight wound, as leaks can lead to many complications. One has the choice of performing the operations sequentially, treating the more pressing condition first, or one may elect to perform the two procedures at the same time. If open-angle glaucoma has been well controlled medically, before cataract extraction, then it usually remains so afterwards. Chronic closed-angle glaucoma is always unpredictable and requires close supervision. Previous drainage surgery makes the cataract extraction more difficult. The two commonest problems are:

(i) The pupil dilates poorly as a result of posterior synechiae.
(ii) The drainage bleb encroaches on to the cornea, forcing the surgeon to place the incision more anteriorly or in a different quadrant of the limbus.

There are specific advantages in removing cataracts in glaucomatous patients. The optic disc is more easily seen, perimetry is more reliable and miotic drops may be used without impairing the visual acuity.

7.1.2.5 Uveitis

Uveitis used to be regarded as a contraindication to IOL implantation but modern techniques and the use of heparin-coated lenses have given excellent results (see Section 7.2.2.2). Provided that the uveitis is under control, the indications for surgery are the same as for the otherwise normal patient. This is a particularly important advance as these patients are relatively young and frequently develop posterior subcapsular opacities, sometimes as a result of the inflammation and sometimes as a result of treatment with corticosteroids. The management of uveitis and cataract in children poses exceptionally difficult problems and these patients are usually treated by paediatric ophthalmologists.

7.1.2.6 Amblyopia

In some cases, there is no doubt that a patient has a well-developed amblyopia. It should be remembered, however, that patients use the term 'lazy eye' to describe both amblyopia and an otherwise normal ametropic eye compared with its emmetropic fellow. If a patient has a manifest squint, it is usually clear from the history whether it is infantile in origin. It is possible, however, that a squint of recent onset arises as a result of cataract development which causes loss of vision and binocularity. In the latter case, the prognosis for the restoration of binocular vision is good. If the squint, which is usually divergent, has a large angle then strabismus surgery may be needed. The two operations can be performed simultaneously.

7.1.2.7 Retinal detachment

If retinal detachment surgery has been successful in an eye which subsequently develops cataract, then surgery is performed in the usual way. If the fellow eye should develop cataract, a careful examination of the retina is essential and any tears or conditions that predispose to retinal detachment should be treated by cryotherapy. Retinal detachment may occur after cataract surgery and this is discussed later (see Section 7.3.5.4).

7.1.2.8 Corneal disorders

Corneal opacities are seen much less frequently since the development of effective antibiotics and antiviral agents. The introduction of seat belts and improved safety standards at work have also reduced the incidence of corneal scarring. If a patient has severe corneal scarring, then one has to decide whether or not to perform a penetrating keratoplasty at the same time as the cataract extraction. A cataract extraction may precipitate endothelial failure in a pre-existing graft but keratoplasty following cataract extraction is usually uncomplicated, as is the combined procedure.

Mild degrees of endothelial dystrophy are common in the elderly population and are not a contraindication to cataract surgery these days.

If the endothelium is very abnormal, then an endothelial cell count is useful to assess the risk of postoperative corneal oedema. The normal cell count is about 2500 per mm^2 and a density of more than 1000 per mm^2 is acceptable.

7.1.2.9 Diabetes mellitus

Diabetes is no longer considered to be a contraindication to IOL implantation. Poorly controlled diabetics are more prone to infections which can be disastrous when they occur within the eye. These days surgery is not performed until the diabetes is properly controlled, and in the rare event of a postoperative infection, we have a range of powerful antibiotics and surgical techniques to deal with endophthalmitis before irreversible damage occurs. This is discussed further under Section 7.3. As in cases of uveitis, there is evidence that the heparin-coated IOL is the lens of choice in the diabetic eye. Cataract surgery may be indicated in diabetics at a relatively early stage in the development of the lens opacity for three reasons:

(a) Diabetics need to read syringes and ampoule labels.
(b) Many diabetics have mobility problems and need to retain a driving licence.
(c) The treatment of diabetic retinopathy has advanced considerably along with the development of modern cataract surgery. The basis of treatment is to apply laser burns to the ischaemic retina in the earliest stages of macular oedema and proliferative retinopathy. To do this successfully, requires relatively clear media enabling satisfactory ophthalmoscopy, fluorescein angiography and the application of the laser burns.

7.2 Operative techniques

7.2.1 Glossary

The techniques of cataract surgery are changing almost daily. The last few years have seen the publication of dozens of books on cataract surgery, there are societies in most developed countries devoted exclusively to discussing cataract techniques and there are several journals also concerned solely with this topic. I shall not attempt a magisterial review of the whole subject but will describe how my colleagues and

I, at Bradford, remove cataracts in 1993 and how we may be removing them in 1994.

New words are continually coined to describe new techniques and some of the older terms can cause confusion. Therefore, I shall start this section with a brief glossary.

An *intracapsular* cataract extraction is the removal of the whole lens including the intact capsule. This operation has now been superseded by the *extracapsular* cataract extraction in which the anterior capsule is opened and the nucleus and cortex are then removed leaving an intact posterior capsule.

The anterior capsule may be opened in several ways. One of the most popular methods used to be the *'beer can' capsulotomy* in which a circle of tiny perforations was made in the anterior capsule and then the central portion could be removed like a circular postage stamp. More recently the capsule has been opened by a curved slit and this has been called an *endocapsular* or *intercapsular extraction*. The most recent advance has been the development of *capsulorhexis* in which a circular tear in the anterior capsule is fashioned of sufficient size to allow delivery of the nucleus.

Phacoemulsification is a means of removing the nucleus by using a hollow needle vibrating at ultrasonic frequencies (45 kHz) to disrupt the densely compacted lens fibres. The microscopic fragments of lens fibres and the surrounding fluid form an emulsion which is aspirated up the hollow needle.

Lensectomy is piecemeal removal of the soft infantile lens, capsule, and, if necessary, anterior vitreous, by an irrigation aspiration system incorporating an oscillating cutter, within the aspirating needle.

An IOL implant consists of an *optic* and a *haptic* which supports the optic. Haptics are usually in the form of open loops but many designs have been produced. These days, haptics are usually made of the same material as the optic such as polymethylmethacrylate(PMMA) or one of the new silicone compounds. Polypropylene has also been widely used.

7.2.2 History

7.2.2.1 Cataract extraction

Modern cataract surgery began on the 29th November 1949 at St. Thomas's Hospital, London, when Harold Ridley, now Sir Harold, removed a cataract by the extracapsular technique and placed an IOL made of PMMA in the posterior chamber. History has proved that Sir Harold chose the correct operation. The same site for placing an implant and the same material is still used today. Although so many of Sir Harold's insights were correct, implant surgery was not widely accepted for almost 30 years. Many surgeons were reluctant to follow Ridley at that time, before the development of microsurgical techniques permitted the use of the extracapsular operation on immature cataracts. Intracapsular extraction was being developed concurrently to deal with the immature cataract problem. The intracapsular operation gave excellent results, particularly with contact lenses. Many surgeons thought that the way forward would be to design IOLs suitable for implantation following intracapsular extraction. The disadvantage of intracapsular extraction is that there is no posterior capsule to support the implant and to prevent vitreous coming forward into the anterior chamber. Choyce [1] devised many anterior chamber lenses with haptics resting in the drainage angle, and Binkhorst [2] devised a lens which was held in place by the sphincter pupillae.

All these lenses had some disadvantages and those of us who implanted the Binkhorst-style lenses were dismayed to find that a significant number of patients suffered corneal decompensation and required corneal grafts. The cause of the decompensation was the extreme mobility of the implant which touched the endothelium during saccades. Pearce reviewed his results with Binkhorst lenses in 1972 [3] and Choyce lenses in 1975 [4]. He decided that the time had come to revisit the extracapsular operation, now performed as a microsurgical procedure on immature cataracts and devised a posterior chamber implant [5]. In the latter half of the 1970s, there was a worldwide surge of interest in extracapsular cataract surgery and posterior chamber lenses, so that within 10 years in the UK and USA the intracapsular operation was all but abandoned.

7.2.2.2 Implant

In parallel with the development of surgical techniques, the implants have been improved both in design and in manufacturing standards. Although an IOL implant appears to be an unsophisticated device, the requirements are formidable. Each lens must be perfectly smooth

and free from internal stresses. Absolute sterility is essential and there must be no residual monomers or dimers left within the implant that could leach out into the eye. Most lenses these days have ultraviolet-absorbing compounds within the PMMA which have proved to be completely safe. Although PMMA is well tolerated within the eye, it has been noted that in some patients, inflammatory deposits form on the implant. Surface-modified lenses are now available such as the heparin-coated lens which, owing to a surface charge effect, is even less reactive than pure PMMA and is used in potentially complicated cases [6].

There has recently been interest shown in bifocal IOLs. Some of these lenses have several concentric optical zones and others use a diffractive system. They appear to work well but the quality of light transmission is inevitably impaired to some extent. They are only of real value if the surgeon can guarantee emmetropia with minimal astigmatism for distance and very few of us have this confidence. In practice, the single-vision implants have a surprisingly good depth of focus, and a VA of $\frac{6}{9}$ and N8 is not uncommon.

In 1967, Kelman [7] devised a machine for phacoemulsification. The earliest machines were bulky and difficult to use and so for nearly 20 years only a few pioneers used this method. Present day machines are now much safer and another revolution in cataract surgery is now well under way. The single greatest advantage of this method of cataract extraction is that it can be performed through a small 3 mm incision. While implants were made of rigid PMMA, with a diameter of 7 mm, there seemed little advantage in performing difficult manoeuvres through a small incision, if it had to be enlarged to allow passage of the implant. Recently, soft foldable implants have become available which can be inserted into the eye through the 3 mm incision. We are now able to perform the whole operation through a small scleral tunnel incision which is self-sealing and therefore requires no sutures and causes no astigmatism.

7.2.3 Preoperative preparations

7.2.3.1 Biometry

The first step in the cataract operation is biometry. In the beginning, standard-power lenses usually of 22.00 D were inserted into the eyes of emmetropic patients and proportional adjustments were made for ametropia. It soon became apparent that many of these patients were left with unacceptable refractive errors, and now the correct power of implant is calculated from the corneal curvature, obtained from keratometry and axial length as determined by ultrasound. The calculations are usually accurate to ± 1.00 D and we usually aim to leave the patient slightly myopic with regular residual astigmatism, the ideal correction being -1.00 DS/$+1.00$ DC $\times$ 90. This degree of ametropia allows reasonable distance and near vision, with uncorrected vision of 6/9 and N8 being obtainable in the best cases.

7.2.3.2 *On the ward*

Immediately before surgery, the pupil is maximally dilated to obtain a perfect view of the lens and its capsule. Sometimes, one has to operate on eyes with pupils that will not dilate and in these circumstances the pupil is dilated or enlarged surgically. In the past, the eyelashes were cut and conjunctival swabs taken but these procedures are no longer considered necessary. Very nervous patients listed for local anaesthesia may be given a mild sedative but we find that full explanations and reassuring nurses are more effective than drugs in allaying fear.

7.2.3.3 *Anaesthesia*

The operation may be performed under either local or general anaesthetic. Most eye surgery throughout the world is performed under local anaesthetic but in the UK we are fortunate to have excellent anaesthetic services in every hospital. Our patients have the choice, except in those circumstances where they are so frail that a general anaesthetic would be unsafe. The instinctive reaction of most patients is to choose general anaesthesia but those who have had the operation on one eye under local and the other under general anaesthesia often prefer the former. Here, there is no pain and no confusion or nausea afterwards. Day case surgery, which is becoming increasingly popular, is usually performed under local anaesthesia.

The aims of local anaesthesia are to prevent pain, abolish the light sense and immobilize the eyeball and eyelids. For many years these aims were achieved by two injections.

(a)   A retrobulbar injection through the skin of the lower eyelid into the muscle cone to block the optic, oculomotor and sensory nerves.

(b)   An injection into the facial nerve as it winds round the neck of the mandible. Recently, it has been shown that injections into the retrobulbar space can damage the optic nerve and perforate the globe in high myopes. Rarely, the anaesthetic agent passes along the sheath of the optic nerve into the cerebrospinal fluid with serious consequences. It has, therefore, been recommended that the nerves within the orbit should be blocked by two peribulbar injections, from which the anaesthetic agent diffuses into the muscle cone in 15 min.

Operative techniques are changing rapidly and so I shall describe the two methods we use in Bradford now, which are also widely used throughout the UK but I suspect that within a year or so this section will appear sadly dated.

7.2.4 The operation

7.2.4.1 *The standard extracapsular extraction*

After sterile drapes have been placed around the eye, a suture is passed through the insertion of the superior rectus to move the eye into the best position in relation to the optical axis of the microscope. The operation can then be performed partly under direct illumination and also by light reflected from the choroid. It is the 'red reflex' that displays the finest details of the lens fibres and capsule and allows the surgeon to remove all lens fibres without damaging the capsule.

Using a diamond knife, a deep groove is cut in the most peripheral region of the cornea, just severing some of the superficial limbal capillaries. The groove extends for 120°, a little more in cataracts with large nuclei.

The anterior chamber is entered at the temporal limit of the groove by a small stab incision, and then Healonid is injected into the anterior chamber. Healonid is one of a group of viscoelastic agents derived from hyaluronic acid (a naturally occurring substance with a molecular weight of more than 10^6 Da). The Healonid protects the corneal endothelium, upon which the transparency of the cornea depends, and maintains the depth of the anterior chamber. A fine hooked needle (a cystitome) is then used to make a tear in the anterior capsule to initiate the capsulorhexis which is completed with a pair of fine forceps. The groove in the cornea is then deepened to become a full thickness incision. In order to assist rotation of the nucleus at a later stage in the operation, saline is injected between the capsule and the cortex (hydrodissection) and between the cortex and the nucleus of the lens (hydrodelamination). These two manoeuvres appear quite spectacular under the microscope. In the first, a reddish wave spreads rapidly from the site of the injection, right around the lens, demonstrating the separation of cortex from capsule. After the second, the nucleus appears to be separated from the cortex by a golden ring. By a combination of tilting and rotation, the nucleus is gently expressed out of the capsular bag, into the anterior chamber and then flushed out of the eye by a gentle stream of saline. The cortex is then removed using an irrigation/aspiration cannula. The irrigating fluid is a balanced saline solution. The cortex can be peeled off the posterior capsule in thin strips and the aim is to remove completely all cortical lens material. Healonid is then injected into the capsular 'bag' and the IOL is passed through the Healonid with care taken to ensure that both haptics are within the capsular bag. The Healonid is then removed from the anterior chamber and the wound sutured with 11/0 Mersilene which is insoluble and, unlike nylon, is not degraded by light. The operation is completed by a subconjunctival injection of antibiotic and steroid. Only the operated eye is padded and the patient returns to the ward.

This operation can be performed on a day case basis but increasing numbers of cataracts are being removed by phacoemulsification. This technique is particularly applicable to day surgery, as the incision is much smaller. It is, therefore, safer and, by careful design of the incision, it is possible to avoid the use of sutures and prevent postoperative astigmatism.

7.2.4.2 *Phacoemulsification*

Phacoemulsification is performed through an oblique incision in the sclera, which enters the anterior chamber just in front of the limbus. The entry incision is 3.2 mm wide which is the correct width to form a watertight seal around the phacoemulsifying irrigation/aspiration probe. Once the incision has been made, the anterior chamber is deepened with a viscoelastic substance such as Healonid and a small capsu-

lorhexis is fashioned. Hydrodissection and hydrodelamination are performed as in the extracapsular technique. The phacoemulsification probe is placed in the anterior chamber and a deep groove sculpted in the nucleus by the rapidly oscillating cutting needle. By a combination of rotating and sculpting, the hard nucleus is completely emulsified and the cortex is then removed as in the standard extracapsular operation. At the present time, we enlarge the wound to 5 mm and insert a rigid PMMA implant. Foldable lenses are being developed, which can be placed in the capsular bag through the 3.2 mm incision, and undoubtedly these will become widely used in the near future. If a self-sealing wound is not used, the wound is closed with one or two nylon sutures and a subconjunctival injection is given as for the extracapsular operation.

At the first dressing, 24 hours after the operation, the eye should be comfortable and the vision should be around 6/18 uncorrected, improving to 6/9 with a pinhole.

Very few restrictions need be placed on patients after cataract surgery but direct trauma to the eye could be catastrophic. For this reason, patients are told to restrict activities so that they are reminded that their eye has undergone major surgery and that complications could occur. One patient expressed this very well when given the list of 'Do's and Don'ts' by replying 'What you are really saying is that I should treasure my eye'.

Patients are given a shield to protect the eye at night and given dark glasses to wear in bright light. Topical steroid and antibiotic drops are prescribed for 4 weeks. Spectacles are usually ordered between 4 and 6 weeks.

7.3 Complications

Complications are rare but cannot be ignored. Millions of cataract operations are performed worldwide every year and inevitably many complications have been recorded. I shall mention only a few of the most important.

7.3.1 Operative

7.3.1.1 *Retrobulbar haemorrhage*

Retrobulbar haemorrhage is due to laceration of the blood vessels during injection of local anaesthetic. The pressure of the ensuing haematoma causes a marked increase in intraocular pressure and the operation has to be abandoned until it is absorbed. Permanent damage to the ocular tissues is exceptionally rare but the blood tracks forwards into the eyelids causing a 'black eye'.

7.3.1.2 Rupture of the posterior capsule

Rupture of the posterior capsule may be associated with forward movement of the vitreous into the anterior chamber, through the incision. Under the most favourable circumstances, the ocular anatomy can be restored, an implant inserted and the visual result can be excellent. If, however, vitreous becomes incarcerated in the wound or mixed with lens protein, the eye becomes chronically inflamed, the macula oedematous and the retina may detach.

7.3.1.3 Expulsive haemorrhage

A very rare, but devastating, complication is expulsive haemorrhage. This is most likely to occur in glaucomatous eyes of elderly atherosclerotic patients. It is due to rupture of the long posterior ciliary arteries when the intraocular pressure suddenly drops as the eye is opened. A small haemorrhage is compatible with the restoration of vision, but, usually, the haemorrhage pushes all the intraocular structures through the incision and the eye is lost. Expulsive haemorrhage may be less likely during phacoemulsification when the intraocular pressure remains at near normal levels.

7.3.2 At 24 hours

At the first dressing the two most important complications are a leaking wound and infection.

7.3.2.1 A leaking wound

A major wound failure is shown by an iris prolapse. The iris tissue is incarcerated in the wound and the pupil is drawn upwards. The patient has to be taken back to theatre for repair of the wound. This complication is now rare as the wound is sutured under high magnification and any imperfect sutures can be replaced. Small leaks can be detected by instilling fluorescein drops when the clear leaking aqueous

contrasts with the tear film. These do not of themselves require treatment.

7.3.2.2 Intraocular infection

Intraocular infection is also rare (<1 in a 1000 cases) but, if not treated immediately, may lead to loss of the eye. In a severe case, the eye is painful and chemosed and the vision poor. Less severe infections may be difficult to diagnose but it is important not to deny the possibility of the infection, as delay in treatment, even by a few hours, can lead to loss of the eye. The basis of the treatment of intraocular infection is a full vitrectomy to remove a good volume of infected material and to obtain adequate tissue and fluid for bacterial culture. Antibiotics are injected into the vitreous cavity and also given systemically. Provided the correct treatment is given without delay, good vision can be restored.

7.3.3 In the first week

7.3.3.1 Late infection

There is still some risk of infection, and patients are asked to report immediately if they think that their vision is deteriorating or the eye is painful. Infections with some bacteria that are part of the normal skin flora (the propionobacter species) tend to be mild but chronic and can pose great difficulties in diagnosis and treatment.

7.3.3.2 Injuries

Occasionally patients sustain a severe injury to the eye in the immediate postoperative period, before the wound is completely healed. These need urgent repair but with microsurgical techniques the results can be surprisingly good.

7.3.4 At 1 month

7.3.4.1 Astigmatism

After the operation, the eye should be white and comfortable with a corrected VA of 6/6 to 6/9. At this stage, the degree of astigmatism is assessed. If there was no preoperative astigmatism, the ideal refraction would be -1.00 DS/$+1.00$ DC $\times 90$. Spectacle corrections of up to 2.50 DC appear to be well tolerated but, above that, steps should be taken to reduce the astigmatism. The most usual form of astigmatism is due to tight sutures which, contrary to what might be expected, steepen the corneal curvature in their own meridian. Thus, a tight suture at 12 o'clock will steepen the cornea along the 90° meridian and require a plus cylinder axis 90 or a minus cylinder axis 180 for correction. A single tight suture could be removed at this stage but it is not safe to remove all the sutures, or a continuous suture until 3 months have elapsed. If the sutures are too lax but the wound is not leaking, it is best to take no action for several months, as the wound may tighten as a result of fibrosis. Occasionally, extra sutures are placed to tighten a wound.

If the vision cannot be improved at 1 month and the media are clear, the cause might be macular oedema. Very mild degrees of macular oedema, as demonstrated by fluorescein angiography, are common, but persistent oedema causing visual loss is unusual ($<1\%$). It is more likely to occur following a complicated operation, especially if the anterior hyaloid face has been ruptured. This is one of the reasons why the extracapsular extraction is preferred to the intracapsular. Anti-inflammatory drugs are given topically and systemically to aid resolution of the oedema but the suspicion is that they do not have a great influence on this particular disorder.

With the use of viscoelastic agents and carefully formulated irrigating solutions, corneal oedema is rare after the insertion of a posterior chamber lens. Indeed, it is surprising how much fluid may pass through the anterior chamber without upsetting the corneal endothelium. Patients who have pre-existing corneal problems, such as Fuch's endothelial dystrophy, may develop corneal oedema which can be persistent. There is no doubt that the iris clip lenses popularized by Binkhorst [2] and Fyodorov [8] were associated with corneal decompensation but this was usually a delayed effect.

7.3.5 Late complications

If the operation and postoperative period have been entirely uncomplicated, then it is our practice to discharge patients to the care of the optometrist and general practitioner at 6 weeks. At this stage they are warned of two minor but frequent complications (approximately 10%) which may occur up to 1–2 years later. These are:

(a) Opacification of the posterior lens capsule;

(b) fragmentation of the sutures giving rise to ocular irritation.

7.3.5.1 Opacification of the lens capsule

Opacification of the capsule is due to regrowth of lens fibres from residual epithelial cells which sometimes undergo metaplasia to fibroblasts. Improvements in lens design have reduced the incidence of capsular opacification but, if it occurs, an Nd:YAG laser is used to cut a central hole in the membrane. This slit-lamp procedure takes only 2–3 min under local anaesthesia. The hole made in the capsule is of the order of 5 mm diameter and does not affect the stability of the implant.

7.3.5.2 Broken sutures

Fragmented sutures are a nuisance to the patient but are easily removed at the slit-lamp. Sometimes, the cause of the persistent irritation in the eye is not recognized and some patients are prescribed antibiotic drops for several weeks before they are referred back for suture removal. If the 'no suture' incisions prove reliable then this complication will fade into history.

7.3.5.3 Glare

In the early days of implant surgery, some patients experienced difficulty with driving at night because the dilated pupil exposed the edge of the implant thereby scattering light. Lens design has improved and surgeons are aware of the importance of placing both haptics in the capsular bag to ensure accurate centration, and so this problem is now less frequent.

7.3.5.4 Retinal detachment

The relationship of cataract extraction to retinal breaks or tears and detachments is complex. Long-term follow up is required to form an accurate picture as detachments may occur several years after cataract surgery. In many cases, the detachment surgeon did not perform the original operation and so essential data might not be available. A recent paper by Davison [9] is particularly valuable, as it records the results of 3120 consecutive cataract extractions performed by a single surgeon, who also treated most of the subsequent retinal breaks and detachments. Although a possible criticism of this paper is that the follow-up period for some patients was only 1 year, there are many valuable points that are worth noting. Estimates of the incidence of detachment following cataract surgery range from 0.02% to 3.60%. In this particular series, there were 25 retinal detachments (0.8%) and 29 (0.9%) retinal tears, a total of 54 retinal break events (RBEs). All the retinal detachments and 25 (86%) of the retinal tears were symptomatic.

The risk factors identified in the Davison [9] study were:

(a) Eyes more than 25 mm long had a 5 times greater chance of developing retinal detachment. Retinal tears were not associated with increased axial length in this series.
(b) Males were 3 times more likely to develop retinal detachment than females [10].
(c) If the fellow eye required treatment for RBE, there was a 40% incidence of RBEs in the now aphakic/pseudophakic eye. Some of these fellow eyes were treated before cataract surgery.
(d) Surgical capsulotomy was associated with a slightly increased incidence of detachment but YAG capsulotomy was not.
(e) Vitreous loss has been associated with detachment in other series but only eight patients in this series had this complication and none developed detachment.

Davison lays great stress on educating his patients to recognize the symptoms of retinal tear and detachment. His patients have a counselling session and video presentation before surgery. One day and 2 weeks after surgery, further advice is given, and follow-up phone calls are also made. As a result of this intensive education, over half of his patients with a retinal break presented before detachment and only two patients failed to regain good sight. It is clear from this report that optometrists have a valuable role in reinforcing the advice given to patients in hospital and in being alert to the possibility that recent floaters, flashing lights and field loss need investigation, particularly if the patient is a male with a long eye.

7.3.5.5 Corneal oedema

Corneal oedema, as a delayed complication, is much less common since the iris clip lenses were abandoned but, if it should occur, the prognosis following penetrating keratoplasty is good. The operation is easier and safer in the presence of an implant and an intact posterior capsule, which prevent forward movement of the vitreous. Modern methods of storing the donor corneas and the organization of the United Kingdom Transplant Service allow the surgeon to schedule the operation on a regular list in the certain knowledge that first-class material will be available.

7.3.5.6 Infection

Delayed infections may occur. In some cases there is a very mild inflammatory reaction that can be partially suppressed by topical steroids. These infections are often due to propionobacter species which adhere to the implant and capsule. Rarely, a severe infection may occur years after surgery, as a result of bacteria gaining access to the anterior chamber along a suture track.

7.4 Results and the future

At least 95% of patients who have no preexisting ocular disease achieve a VA of 6/9 or better. As a consequence of these excellent results, which are well known to the general public, the incidence of cataract surgery is rising steeply in the First and Second Worlds.

In Bradford, we perform 1000 cataract operations a year which is two per thousand of the population per annum. This is nearly double the rate of a decade ago, but in the USA the rate is nearly five per thousand of the population per annum. The reason for this sharp rise is, in part, the increasing proportion of the elderly in the population and also the safety and excellent visual results achieved by modern surgery, which justifies the removal of very early lens opacities. There is some evidence that the high operation rates in the USA arise from dealing with the backlog of patients formerly considered unsuitable for surgery. In future, the rate may settle at around 3.5 to 4.0 per 1000 of the population per annum, if there is no progress in the prevention, or medical treatment, of cataract.

In the Third World, the implications of these figures are awesome. Already millions of people are blind due to cataract and many millions more could benefit from surgery. Those who allocate funds for medical services are faced with increasing demands for this operation. When performed as an inpatient procedure under general anaesthetic, the operation is expensive, but recent advances in 'small wound no suture' surgical techniques make day case surgery safer. There is every prospect that the present high cost of the instrumentation and implants will fall as research and development costs are recouped.

The next step forward in cataract surgery will probably be the development of lasers to emulsify the cataract within the intact capsule. The emulsified material could then be aspirated through a very fine needle and replaced by a plastic material, which would have the physical properties of natural lens protein thereby restoring active accommodation.

The development of cataract surgery has been a tribute to the ingenuity of surgeons, engineers and chemists throughout the world. In this brief review, I have mentioned only a few surgeons who have influenced surgical practice in the UK.

References

1. Choyce, D.P. All acrylic anterior chamber lens implants in ophthalmic surgery. *Lancet*, **ii**, 165–171 (1961)
2. Binkhorst, C.D. Iris supported artificial pseudophakia. A new development in intraocular artificial lens surgery. *Transactions of the Ophthalmological Society of the UK*, **79**, 569–584 (1959)
3. Pearce, J.L. Long term results of the Binkhorst iris clip lens in senile cataract. *British Journal of Ophthalmology*, **59**, 319 (1972)
4. Pearce, J.L. Long term results of the Choyce anterior chamber lens implants Marks V, VI and VII. *British Journal of Ophthalmology*, **59**, 99 (1975)
5. Pearce, J.L. New lightweight sutured posterior chamber lens implants. *Transactions of the Ophthalmological Society*, **96**, 8 (1976)
6. Steinkogler, F.J., Huber, E., Aichmair, M. *et al.* Heparin surface modified PMMA lenses in a prospective double blind study. *European Journal of Implant and Refractive Surgery*, **4**, 79–82 (1992)
7. Kelman, C.D. Phacoemulsification and aspiration. *American Journal of Ophthalmology*, **64**, 23 (1967)
8. Fyodorov, S.N. Long term results of 2000 operations of implantation of the Fyodorov intraocular lens performed in the Soviet Union. *American Intraocular Implant Society Journal*, **3**, 101 (1977)
9. Davison, J.A. Retinal tears and detachments after extracapsular surgery. *Journal of Cataract and Refractive Surgery*, **14**, 624–632 (1988)
10. Bedrick, J.J. Correlation of aphakic retinal detachment and refractive error with gender. *American Journal of Ophthalmology*, **90**, 540–544 (1980)

Recommended reading

A Colour Atlas of Lens Implantation (edited by S.P.B. Percival), Wolfe Publishing Ltd, London (1991)
Paediatric Cataract in the special issue of the *European Journal of Implant and Refractive Surgery*, **2** (4) (December 1990)

8

Spectacle correction

William A. Douthwaite and Alan H. Tunnacliffe

8.1 Optical correction of the aphakic eye

Removal of the crystalline lens results in the condition called aphakia. This may be recognized by: the deep appearance of the anterior chamber; iris tremor and trauma; the loss of two Purkinje images; and remnants of the lens capsule observed by ophthalmoscopy. The surgery required for lens removal often induces astigmatism in the order of 2.00 D, but, the main optical change is due to the removal of an optical component of power around ± 20.00 D. Thus, a previously emmetropic eye becomes highly hyperopic with no ability to accommodate. The eye may be corrected optically using:

(a)   a spectacle lens correction;
(b)   a contact lens correction;
(c)   an intraocular lens (IOL).

The study of the human visual system, in general, attracts workers from a number of scientific disciplines. The list includes biochemists, anatomists, physiologists, psychologists, physicists, ophthalmologists as well as optometrists. It is, however, the area of visual optics and the correction of optical errors where the optometrist has no rival and should have no equal. Sadly, this is the very area that many optometrists find mundane when compared with aspects such as disease detection or the monitoring of the physiological changes induced by contact lens wear. We therefore make no apology for the detail included in this chapter which deals with the optical correction of the aphakic eye by spectacle lenses. There is a considerable amount of published material dealing with this form of optical correction and there are a number of lens designs derived specifically for this problem. This may seem inappropriate when increasing numbers of aphakic patients are corrected by IOLs. There are, however, still circumstances when a spectacle lens may be the only option, and the optometrist must be able to deal with these increasingly rare cases when she or he encounters such a patient. The topics that are investigated also apply to any moderate to high hyperope and are not confined to the aphakic patient exclusively.

8.2 The crystalline lens

Before considering the methods of correcting aphakia, it may be appropriate to examine the crystalline lens itself. From an optical point of view, the complex refractive index changes in the lens make a simplified representation essential. Gullstrand represented the lens in his number 1 schematic eye as shown in Figure 8.1. It can be seen that this schematic lens has a homogeneous nucleus of refractive index 1.406 surrounded by a cortex of refractive index 1.386. The radius of curvature of the anterior and posterior surfaces are 10 mm and -6 mm respectively, with those of the nucleus being 7.91 mm and -5.76 mm.

The axial centre thicknesses are 2.419 mm for the nucleus and 3.6 mm for the whole lens. The

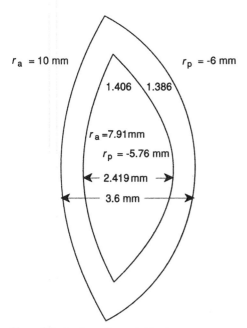

Figure 8.1. A schematic crystalline lens.

equivalent power of this lens is $+19.11$ D with the first and second principal planes being 2.08 mm and 2.205 mm from the anterior pole of the lens, which is 3.6 mm from the anterior corneal vertex.

8.3 Astigmatism

Measurements suggest that the crystalline lens tends to produce against-the-rule astigmatism. This is most likely to be due to:

(a) astigmatic lens surfaces;
(b) lateral displacement of the lens;
(c) lens tilt.

If the crystalline lens is tilted with respect to the visual axis, a 14° tilt is required to produce around 0.50 D of lenticular astigmatism. A 14° tilt is considerably larger than the tilt present in the typical eye and so lenticular astigmatism arising from this source is likely to be very small indeed.

The astigmatism induced by the postoperatively deformed cornea decreases in the first few months after the cataract operation. The changes are largely determined by the choice of material for the sutures and their tightness.

The post-cataract correction is clearly related to the previous refractive state of the eye but this is not the only determining factor. In fact, the relationship between the post-cataract spectacle correction and the previous spectacle correction shows a spread around 3.00 D to 5.00 D on either side of the mean.

8.4 Spectacle correction

The equivalent power of the aphakic eye is that of the cornea alone. The principal points of the typical cornea very nearly coincide with each other and with the vertex of its front surface. Thus, the aphakic eye can be regarded as having only one refracting surface, the power of which can be deduced with reasonable accuracy using the keratometer. The drastic reduction in the converging power of the eye produces an ocular refraction of $+13.00$ D in the Gullstrand–Emsley schematic eye which would require a spectacle lens power of $+11.31$ D at a vertex distance of 12 mm.

In the Gullstrand simplified eye (made aphakic) the parameters are as illustrated in Figure 8.2. The space occupied by the lens is filled with aqueous and we can now assume a single homogeneous medium of refractive index 1.336. If an eye has an axial length 24.17 mm with a cornea of radius of curvature 7.8 mm, we can calculate the ocular refraction as follows. The light rays within the eye in Figure 8.2 emerge from the corneal surface with a vergence ② of 1336/24.17 which is $+55.275$ D if the light rays are to focus on the retina. The power of the single refracting surface is 336/7.8 which is

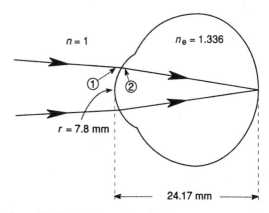

Figure 8.2. The Gullstrand simplified eye made aphakic. ① and ② represent the respective incident and emergent vergences on the corneal surface. The light rays are assumed to be paraxial.

+43.077 D. The incident vergence on the corneal surface ① must be

55.275 − 43.077 = ocular refraction
$$= +12.198 \text{ D}$$

As a cross-check for this result we can see that an incident vergence of +12.198 D on a surface of power +43.077 D results in an emergent vergence which is the algebraic addition of these values and this comes to +55.275 D which is the dioptric length of the eye. The +12.198 D is considerably less than the 20.00 D power of the crystalline lens. The difference is due to the effectivity of measuring the refractive change at the cornea.

If we go on to correct this eye with a spectacle lens (assumed to be thin) at a vertex distance of 12 mm, the power of this lens can be calculated as follows using the step along method and Figure 8.3. We have already deduced that the ocular refraction is +12.198 D. This is the vergence ③ in Figure 8.3. The reciprocal of this vergence gives the distance CF′ in metres. If we add on the vertex distance we have distance SF′. The reciprocal of this distance gives us vergence ② which is equal to the power of the spectacle lens F_s. Thus:

Vergence (D)		Distance (mm)
③ = +12.198	→ $\dfrac{1000}{12.198}$ →	81.98 = CF′
		12.00 (add)
		————
② = +10.64	← $\dfrac{1000}{93.98}$ ←	93.98 = SF′
———		
① = +00.00		

$F_s = +10.64$ This is the back vertex power (BVP) of a thick or thin lens.

If the subject was myopic by an amount around 10.00 to 12.00 D in their youth, they would be near emmetropic after a cataract operation. Obviously, hyperopic subjects with cataract will be more hyperopic than the +12.198 D calculated above for the Gullstrand eye, after removal of the crystalline lens.

8.5 Precautions to be taken when refracting the aphakic eye

A number of precautions need to be considered when the optometrist is refracting a moderate to high hyperope. The problems are further compounded in the case of the aphakic patient because of the absence of accommodation. The precautions worth considering are listed below.

(a) Retinoscopy may best be carried out with positive cylinders. This minimizes the spherical power required for correction. Also, reference to the retinoscopy equations shows that the speed of the reflex movement is slower for a positive error than that of a negative error of the same power. Thus, theoretically, the use of positive cylinders improves the sensitivity of the retinoscopy technique.

(b) The number of lenses in the trial frame must be kept to a minimum and the most powerful lenses must be placed in the rear cells of the trial frame with the weakest lenses in the front. This ensures that the algebraic addition of the lenses will give a

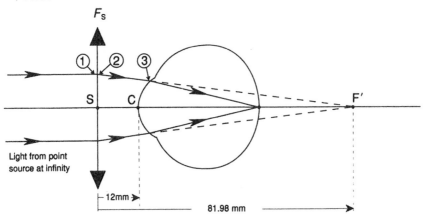

Figure 8.3. The relationship between the ocular and spectacle refraction. Once again the light rays are assumed to be paraxial and the numbers enclosed in the circles identify the vergences.

power nearly equal to the BVP of the lens combination. Even so, the only way of measuring the true BVP is to place the combination of lenses in the trial frame in a focimeter.

(c) The effective power of the spectacle lens at the eye will be greater than its BVP. This means that a $+0.25$ D power change at the spectacle plane will produce a power change greater than $+0.25$ D at the eye. Thus, the optometrist must consider this point when deciding on the level of precision to adopt during the refractive routine. It must also be noted that the absence of the facility for accommodation means that, if the cylindrical lens is made less positive during the subjective assessment of astigmatism, the sphere must be made more positive by half the power change in the cylinder.

(d) The vertex distance must be kept to a minimum. This is achieved when the back surface of the rearmost lens is just clearing the eye lashes. The vertex distance is the distance from this back surface to the anterior corneal vertex, and this must be measured. There are a number of advantages to keeping the vertex distance small and they are listed below. A fuller explanation of these features is given in later sections of this chapter.

   (i) The fields of vision (both the static and the motor fields) are maximal. This is particularly important because the high plus lenses restrict the field of view of the wearer, producing a ring scotoma and this can be one of the most difficult aspects to adapt to.

   (ii) The spectacle magnification is minimized, which again may help ease the adaptation problems of the wearer. The magnification of the eye behind the lens is also minimized which helps to produce a better cosmetic appearance.

   (iii) For any given angular rotation of the eye, the region of the lens used to form a retinal image will be less eccentric with a small vertex distance. This means that the peripheral aberrations of the spectacle lens are kept to a minimum because these

aberrations (oblique astigmatism, curvature, distortion and transverse chromatic aberration) all increase as the more peripheral regions of the lens are used.

   (iv) The mean oblique image vergence, when looking at a near object, may be different from that of a paraxial pencil of light rays. Once again the difference between the paraxial and oblique rays increases with eccentricity, requiring the wearer to move the near work further away when using the peripheral regions of the lens. The small vertex distance means that for any given angular rotation of the eye, the region of the lens used is nearer the paraxial region.

(e) The near-vision effectivity of the trial lens and the prescription lens are likely to be different (particularly with reduced aperture trial lenses). This means that typically $+0.50$ D should be added to the reading addition found at the time of the refraction.

(f) Any binocular measurements will require the trial lenses to be accurately centred in order to avoid any unwanted prism. An error of 1 mm in centration will induce a prism over 1Δ. Indeed the centration must be accurate when making monocular measurements because there is an implied assumption when performing refractions and dispensing corrections that the eye looks through the optical centre of the spectacle lens, with the lens optical axis running through the eye's centre of rotation. The optometrist must also remember to alter the centration distance of the lenses, when moving from distance vision assessment to near, to compensate for the convergence of the visual axes. It may also be worth considering altering the angle of side of the trial frame (to alter the pantoscopic angle) and the bridge height to compensate for the depression of the visual axes, again to ensure that the optical axis of the spectacle lens passes through the eye's centre of rotation in the vertical plane.

(g) Refractive complications can arise as a result of factors such as pupil size and shape, pupil position, vitreous movement and lens capsule changes. In the case of the young aphake, the visual development may be abnormal and therefore amblyopia and binocular vision problems may become apparent after the operation.

8.6 The retinal image size in aphakia

In Gullstrand's simplified schematic eye, the cornea is considered to be a single surface and the crystalline lens to be a homogeneous structure with two surfaces (see Figure 8.4) giving surface powers in the eye of $+7.70\,D$ and $+12.83\,D$ for the anterior and posterior lens surfaces respectively. It will be assumed that the aphakic eye is like the eye in Figure 8.4 without the lens.

8.7 The image size in the simplified eye

The retinal image in this eye is produced by the three refracting surfaces shown in Figure 8.5, which illustrates the path of light rays from the top of a distant object standing on the optical axis. Thus, the distant object subtends a visual angle θ.

$h_1' = f_1 \tan \theta$

h_1' becomes the object for surface 2 and the image produced by surface 2 is h_2'; therefore magnification

$$m_2 = \frac{h_2'}{h_1'}$$

$$= \frac{h_2'}{f_1 \tan \theta}$$

therefore $h_2' = f_1 \tan \theta . m_2$

h_2' becomes the object for surface 3 and the image produced by surface 3 is h_3'; therefore magnification

$$m_3 = \frac{h_3'}{h_2'}$$

$$= \frac{h_3'}{f_1 \tan \theta . m_2}$$

therefore $h_3' = f_1 \tan \theta . m_2 . m_3$

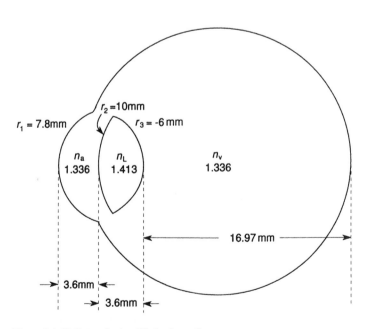

Figure 8.4. Gullstrands simplified schematic eye.

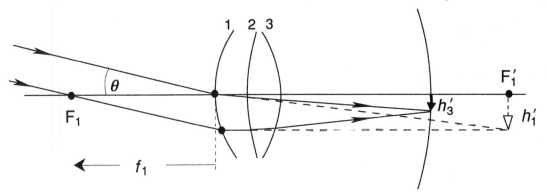

Figure 8.5. Image size produced by three refracting surfaces.

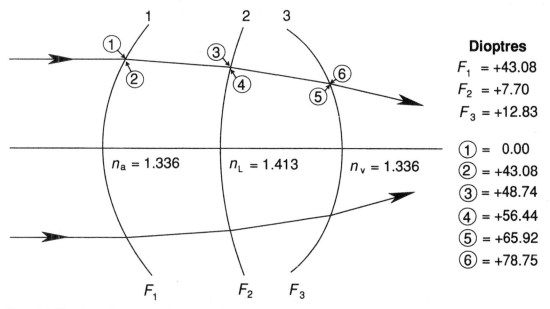

Dioptres

F_1 = +43.08
F_2 = +7.70
F_3 = +12.83

① = 0.00
② = +43.08
③ = +48.74
④ = +56.44
⑤ = +65.92
⑥ = +78.75

Figure 8.6. The change in vergence through the three surface system.

But magnification = $\dfrac{\text{image size}}{\text{object size}}$

$= \dfrac{\text{object vergence}}{\text{image vergence}}$

From Figure 8.6 we can see that

$m_2 = \dfrac{③}{④}$ (magnification due to surface 2)

and that

$m_3 = \dfrac{⑤}{⑥}$ (magnification due to surface 3)

Therefore

$h_3' = f_1 \tan \theta . \dfrac{③}{④} . \dfrac{⑤}{⑥}$

In this case

$f_1 = \dfrac{1}{-F_1}$

and

$F_1 = \dfrac{(n-1)}{r}$

$= \dfrac{336}{7.8} = +43.08 \text{ D}$

$$f_1 = \frac{1000}{-43.08} = -23.21 \text{ mm}$$

Vergence (D)	Distance (mm)
② $= +43.081 \rightarrow \dfrac{336}{43.08} \rightarrow 31.01$	
	3.6 (subtract)
③ $= +48.74 \leftarrow \dfrac{336}{27.41} \leftarrow 27.41$	
$F_2 = +7.7$	
④ $= +56.441 \rightarrow \dfrac{413}{56.44} \rightarrow 25.04$	
	3.6 (subtract)
⑤ $= +65.921 \leftarrow \dfrac{413}{21.44} \leftarrow 21.44$	
$F_3 = +12.83$	
⑥ $= +78.75$	

therefore

$$h_3' = -23.21 \tan\theta \cdot \frac{48.74}{56.44} \cdot \frac{65.92}{78.75}$$

$$= -16.78 \tan\theta = h_e' \text{ (retinal image size in the emmetropic eye).}$$

Figure 8.7 illustrates the path of light rays for the corrected aphakic eye.

h_3' CORRECTED:

$$h_3' = f_1 \tan\theta \, \frac{③}{④} \cdot \frac{⑤}{⑥}$$

$$= \frac{-1000}{F_1} \tan\theta \cdot \frac{③}{④} \cdot \frac{⑤}{⑥}$$

Calculation of the vergences

axial length of the eye $= 24.17$ mm

therefore vergence ⑥ must be

$$\frac{1336}{24.17} = +55.28 \text{ D}$$

power of eye's reduced surface

$$F_c = \frac{336}{7.8} = +43.08 \text{ D}$$

We will use a correcting spectacle lens set at a vertex distance of 12 mm which has a plano back surface, a central thickness of 10.67 mm and a refractive index of 1.523.

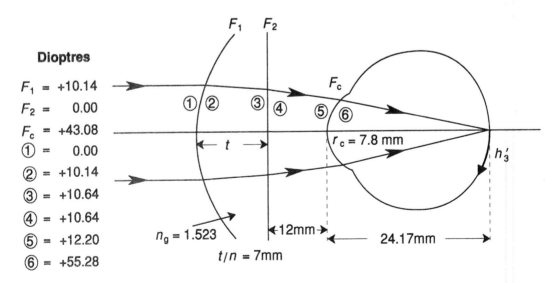

Dioptres	
$F_1 =$	$+10.14$
$F_2 =$	0.00
$F_c =$	$+43.08$
① $=$	0.00
② $=$	$+10.14$
③ $=$	$+10.64$
④ $=$	$+10.64$
⑤ $=$	$+12.20$
⑥ $=$	$+55.28$

F_1 F_2

F_c

$r_c = 7.8$ mm

h_3'

$n_g = 1.523$

$\leftarrow$ 12mm $\rightarrow$

$\leftarrow$ 24.17mm $\rightarrow$

$t/n = 7$mm

Figure 8.7. The path of the light rays in the corrected aphakic eye.

Vergence (D)   Distance (mm)

⑥ = +55.28

F_c = +43.08   (subtract)

⑤ = +12.20 → $\dfrac{1000}{12.28}$ → 81.97

                 12   (add)

④ = +10.64 ← $\dfrac{1000}{93.97}$ ← 93.97

F_2 =   00.00   (subtract)

③ = +10.64 → $\dfrac{1523}{10.64}$ → 143.14

             7   add $\dfrac{t}{n}$

② = +10.14 ← $\dfrac{1523}{150.14}$ ← 150.14

① = +00.00   (subtract)

F_1 = +10.14   and $\dfrac{1000}{10.14}$ = 98.62 mm

therefore

h_3' = −98.62 tan θ . $\dfrac{10.64}{10.64} \cdot \dfrac{12.20}{55.28}$

   = −21.76 tan θ = h_c' (retinal image size corrected)

$\dfrac{\text{aphakic retinal image size corrected}}{\text{emmetropic aphakic retinal image size}}$

$= \dfrac{-21.76 \tan \theta}{-16.78 \tan \theta} = 1.297$

Therefore, the image in the aphakic eye is 29.7% larger than that in the emmetropic eye. The patient must adapt to this vastly increased retinal image size. Distance judgement is particularly affected with objects appearing to be nearer than they are. There are other problems that require adaptation and these will be discussed later in the chapter.

8.8 Spectacle magnification

The spectacle magnification can be defined as:

$\dfrac{h_c'}{h_u'} = \dfrac{\text{retinal image size in the corrected eye}}{\text{retinal image size in the uncorrected eye}}$

The increase in the retinal image size due to the correcting lens arises from two factors:

(a) the power factor;
(b) the shape factor.

The total spectacle magnification is the power factor multiplied by the shape factor. The power factor is the magnification of the retinal image due to the lens being a finite distance from the eye's entrance pupil. The shape factor is the magnification of the retinal image due to the lens being a thick lens of a specified form.

8.8.1 Power factor

Figure 8.8 illustrates a thin correcting spectacle lens positioned at a finite distance from the eye.

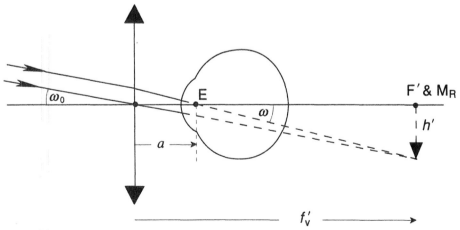

Figure 8.8. The effect of vertex distance on the size of the retinal image. E represents the position of the eyes entrance pupil.

The distant object being viewed is standing on the axis of the system and subtends an angle ω_0 at the spectacle plane. If the eye were removed from the diagram, this lens would form an image h' in the focal plane of the lens. The light ray illustrated is coming from the top of the object and passes through the optical centre of the lens and continues undeviated to emerge at an angle ω_0 to the optical axis. However, when the eye is present as shown in the diagram, h' becomes the object for the eye since it is in the far point plane through M_R. Thus the corrected visual angle is ω where ω is the angle subtended by h' at E the entrance pupil of the eye.

$$\text{Spectacle magnification} = \frac{\omega}{\omega_0}$$

$$\tan \omega_0 = \frac{-h'}{f_v'} \quad \text{(negative sign required for inverted image)}$$

$$\tan \omega = \frac{-h'}{f_v' - a}$$

where a is the distance from the lens to the entrance pupil of the eye. Thus

$$\text{spectacle magnification} = \frac{-h'/(f_v' - a)}{-h'/f_v'}$$

$$= \frac{f_v'}{f_v' - a}$$

$$= \frac{1}{1 - aF_v'}$$

where F_v' is the BVP of the spectacle lens and a is the distance from the back vertex of the lens to the entrance pupil of the eye (in metres).

The value $\dfrac{1}{1 - aF_v'}$ is called the *power factor*.

8.8.2 Shape factor

If we assume in Figure 8.9 that the spectacle lens is thin and of focal length f_v', then we can see that the image size at the far point of the eye is h_1'. However, the thick and possibly curved spectacle lens will behave like an equivalent thin lens placed at P' of focal length f' (the equivalent focal length). Thus the spectacle lens actually produces an image size h_2'. The ratio of

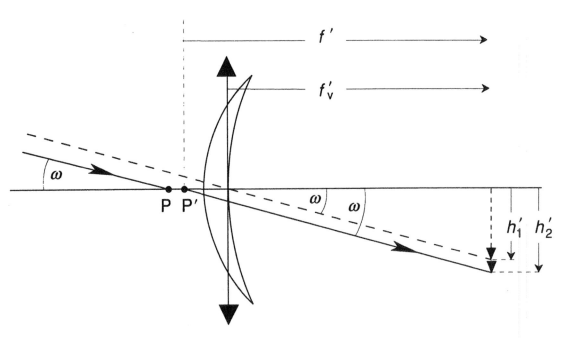

Figure 8.9. The effect of lens form on image size. h_1' and h_2' are the image sizes produced by a thin lens with the same power as the BVP of the thick lens. The distant object stands on the optical axis and subtends an angle ω.

these two image sizes is called the *shape factor*.

Shape factor $= \dfrac{h_2'}{h_1'}$

$\tan \omega = \dfrac{-h_1'}{f_v'}$

and $\tan \omega = \dfrac{-h_2'}{f'}$

therefore

shape factor $= \dfrac{-f' \tan \omega}{-f_v' \ \tan \omega}$

$= \dfrac{f'}{f_v'}$

If these distances are expressed in metres, then their reciprocals give the lens power in dioptres.

Thus shape factor $= \dfrac{F_v' =}{F_e}$

where F_v' is the BVP and F_e is the power of the equivalent thin lens at P′.

The BVP of a thick lens

$$F_v' = \dfrac{F_1 + F_2 - [(t/n)F_1 . F_2]}{1 - (t/n)F_1}$$

and the equivalent power
$F_e = F_1 + F_2 - [(t/n)F_1 . F_2]$
where F_1 is the front surface power, F_2 is the back surface power and t/n is the reduced thickness of the lens.

Therefore shape factor $= \dfrac{1}{1 - (t/n)F_1}$

N.B. Increasing F_1 or t will make the shape factor larger, which produces a larger corrected retinal image size.

8.8.3 Spectacle magnification

The spectacle magnification (SM) will be the product of the power factor and the shape factor. Thus

$$SM = \left(\dfrac{1}{1 - aF_v'}\right)\left(\dfrac{1}{1 - (t/n)F_1}\right)$$

8.9 Correction by spectacles

The magnified retinal image produced when the aphakic eye is corrected by a spectacle lens is

just one of the many problems that the aphakic patient has to face. One other major problem arises from the fact that the correcting lens is of high power and is therefore more likely to suffer from optical aberrations. The most noticeable aberration for the wearer of this type of lens is oblique astigmatism. Less noticeable effects arise as a result of field curvature, distortion and transverse chromatic aberration (TCA). The only variable available to the lens designer, apart from the characteristics of the lens material, is the lens form, i.e. the lens can be manufactured steeper or flatter. There is also the option of replacing the spherical surfaces with aspherical ones.

Table 8.1 illustrates the effect of lens form on a +6.00 D spheric lens when the eye rotates 30° to look through the peripheral region of the lens. The centre of rotation of the eye is 27 mm from the back vertex of the lens which is made of glass of refractive index 1.523 and V value (constringence) 59. Table 8.1 illustrates that form has a significant effect on oblique gaze focus, with the final form in the Table eliminating oblique astigmatism, giving minimum distortion and TCA but producing a thicker lens. Spectacle lenses for aphakia have always been a challenge for lens designers since the problems found with lower-power lenses are simply accentuated. The optical problem of oblique astigmatism in aphakia resulted in a compromise solution until the advent of relatively inexpensive aspherical surfaces. Three decades ago we kept weight and thickness to a minimum by using small eye sizes or lenticulars with spherical surfaces. Now we have lenses with aspherical surfaces made in CR39 material which solve or lessen the impact of the problems.

The problems associated with spectacle lenses for aphakia are:

(a) weight and thickness;
(b) oblique gaze performance;
(c) magnification;
(d) lack of accommodation;

TABLE 8.1 The effect of form on lens performance (data for a 30° rotation and spheric form)

Back surface power (D)	Oblique power (D)	Distortion (%)	TCA	tc (mm)
0.00	+6.22/+1.37	8.92	0.20	6.68
−3.75	+5.83/+0.36	6.26	0.19	6.94
−7.12	+5.65/ 0.00	4.76	0.19	7.51

(e) field of view;
(f) vertical and horizontal centration;
(g) protection from UV radiation.

These topics are discussed individually in the remainder of this chapter.

8.9.1 Weight and thickness

In order to minimize weight and thickness we must consider the materials currently available for lens manufacture. These are listed in Tables 8.2 and 8.3. Note that the relative curvature is the ratio of the refractivity $(n - 1)$ of Spectacle Crown divided by that of the high-index material. This gives an approximate indication of the fractional reduction in centre thickness compared with that of a Crown glass lens.

Obviously, the use of lower refractive index materials will result in greater lens centre thickness but the weight of the lens may still be

TABLE 8.2 Properties of high-index glasses compared with 1.523 Spectacle Crown

Supplier	Index	V value	Specific gravity	Relative curvature
ALL				
Crown	1.523	58.9	2.54	1.00
CORNING				
Low-mass crown	1.523	53.0	2.38	1.00
PILKINGTON				
Slimline 640	1.600	41.0	2.58	0.87
CORNING				
Titanium 1.6	1.600	41.4	2.60	0.87
DESAG				
Hi-Crown 42	1.604	41.8	2.67	0.87
SCHOTT				
S.1018	1.601	42.2	2.67	0.87
Highlite	1.701	31.0	2.99	0.75
PILKINGTON				
Slimline 730	1.700	30.0	2.99	0.75
Slimline 750	1.700	50.8	3.38	0.75
SCHOTT				
Tital 40	1.701	39.5	3.20	0.75
CORNING				
Titanium	1.701	41.5	3.16	0.75
HOYA				
LHI	1.702	40.2	2.99	0.75
DESAG				
Lantal	1.800	35.4	3.62	0.65
CORNING				
Lanthanum	1.804	34.7	3.66	0.65
HOYA				
THI-II	1.806	33.3	3.47	0.65
NIKON				
Pointal	1.830	32.0	3.59	0.63

TABLE 8.3 Properties of plastics materials

Plastics	Index	V value	Specific gravity	Relative curvature
PPGI*				
CR-39	1.498	58.0	1.32	1.05
SIGNET AR-MORLITE				
RLX Lite	1.556	37.7	1.21	0.93
YOUNGER				
Lite	1.556	37.7	1.22	0.93
HOYA				
HL-II	1.560	40.0	1.27	0.93
NIKON				
LiteDXII	1.560	41.0	1.17	0.93
Lite II	1.580	34.5	1.47	0.90
Lite III	1.600	36.0	1.34	0.87
GENTEX				
Polycarb.	1.586	30.0	1.20	0.89
PRIMLANDS				
TFE 160	1.594	35.7	1.34	0.88
NORVILLE				
Norlite 1.60	1.600	30.0	1.38	0.87
PENTAX				
Superthin 1.6	1.600	36.0	1.34	0.87
SEIKO				
Super 16	1.600	34.0	1.38	0.87
TORAY				
Uvithin & TL 160†	1.609	32.0	1.41	0.86

*Pittsburgh Plate Glass Industries.
†Saffron and Essilor names.

low because of the low specific gravity. Lens thickness is also influenced by the lens design and this is illustrated in Table 8.4. Notice in the Table how the aspheric lenticular is slightly thinner than the spheric lenticular and is more than 2.50 D flatter. This latter point means the lens appears to bulge noticeably less and is therefore better cosmetically.

8.9.2 Oblique gaze performance

Lens designers have sought to perfect the aspheric lens because of the poor performance of spheric lenses for the aphakic eye. High-powered plus spheric lenses, above about + 7.50 D, cannot fully correct oblique astigmatism. Aspheric lenses can do this and at the same time reduce distortion and TCA.

8.9.2.1 Oblique astigmatism and mean oblique error

Figure 8.10 illustrates the fundamental principles and the terminology. For an ocular rotation θ, the pencil of light rays passes through the eye with the chief ray of the pencil passing

TABLE 8.4 Thicknesses of three best form CR-39 lenses of +12.00 power

Form	Back surface power (D)	Edge thickness (mm)	Front surface power (D)	Centre thickness (mm)
50 mm full aperture	−5.00	1.5	+15.27	9.98
40 mm spheric lenticular	−5.00	3 at 40 mm	+15.59	8.00
40 mm aspheric lenticular	−2.00	3 at 40 mm	+13.06	7.66

through the eye's centre of rotation. It can be seen that the light emerging from the lens forms an astigmatic pencil resulting in a horizontal (tangential) line focus and a vertical (sagittal) line focus with the disc of least confusion between the two. An 'ideal' lens would produce a single point image which would coincide with the far point sphere.

Distance $QT = f_t'$ Distance $QS = f_s'$

$$\frac{1}{f_t'} = F_t \qquad \frac{1}{f_s'} = F_s$$

Oblique astigmatic error (OAE) = $F_t - F_s$

Mean oblique power (MOP) = $\dfrac{F_t + F_s}{2}$

Mean oblique error (MOE) = MOP − BVP

The problem with a spherical surface receiving an oblique pencil of rays is that it introduces an asymmetrical refraction in the tangential meridian compared with that of the sagittal meridian. If the asymmetry introduced at the first surface can be cancelled by the asymmetry introduced at the second surface, the oblique rays will form a point focus along the chief ray and the oblique astigmatism is eliminated. This cannot be achieved using spherical surfaces for typical aphakic corrections. Note that oblique powers are measured at the vertex sphere in order to allow a direct comparison with the paraxial BVP of

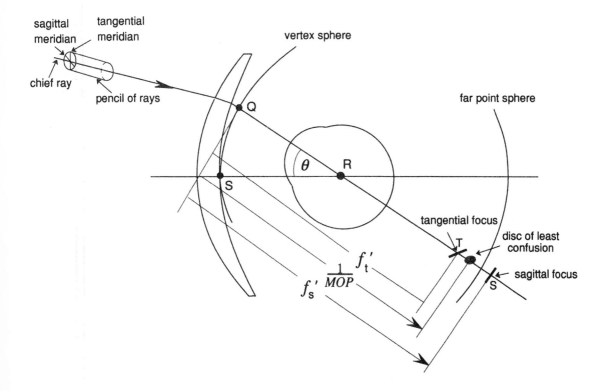

Figure 8.10. The astigmatic line foci and the disc of least confusion formed by an oblique pencil of rays. R is the centre of rotation of the eye. Note that the radius of the vertex sphere is SR and the radius of the far point sphere is the distance from the far point to point R.

the lens. The 'ideal' lens mentioned above would be a lens where

$$F_t = F_s = \text{BVP}$$

This results in a point image being formed on the far point sphere. The concept of the vertex sphere also ensures that the power is always measured at the same distance from the corneal vertex no matter in which direction the eye is looking.

It is still possible to have zero oblique astigmatism and yet have a power error. The MOE will be zero only when the mean oblique power equals the lens BVP. So the 'ideal' lens is one where the oblique astigmatism is zero and the mean oblique error is zero for all directions and degrees of gaze.

8.9.2.2 Aspheric lenses for aphakia

The ideal of zero oblique astigmatism can be achieved by using a prolate ellipsoid for the front surface of the lens (see Figure 8.11.) This is possible because, except at the vertex, an ellipsoidal surface is astigmatic. This astigmatism can be used to help cancel the astigmatism due to the asymmetry of oblique refraction which adds to the advantages we have already seen, namely that aspheric lenticulars are flatter and thinner than an equivalent spheric lenticu-

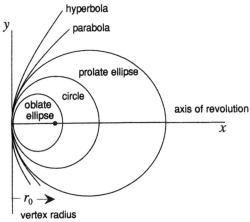

	$p > 1$	oblate ellipse
	$p = 1$	circle
The conicoid equation	$0 < p < 1$	prolate ellipse
$y^2 = 2r_0 x - p x^2$	$p = 0$	parabola
	$p < 0$	hyperbola

Figure 8.11. Conicoids. Note particularly the prolate (flattening) ellipse which is used in the example in the text.

lar. However, when oblique astigmatism is eliminated there will still be an MOE. Taking the $+12.00$ D aspheric example of Table 8.4 which has a p value of 0.6 and a back surface power of -2.00 D, the MOP is $+11.57$ D so the MOE is $+11.57 - 12.00 = -0.43$ D. This calculation is for an ocular rotation of 30° and a distant object. In fact this particular lens design produces 0.25 D of OAE in these circumstances. It is in fact possible to choose a p value and back surface power to make the OAE zero but the MOE increases to -0.66 D. The spheric lenticular from Table 8.4 in comparison produces 1.17 D of OAE and a MOE of $+0.45$ D. In both lenses, the performance improves as the ocular rotation decreases.

The flatter lens form of the aspheric design is cosmetically advantageous, and, with the advent of computer-controlled surface generators, a further improvement in cosmesis is possible. Lens designers have been able to use higher order curves than the second order conicoids. These latest curves are polynomials where the sagitta x of the front aspherical surface is expressed in terms of the chord semidiameter y by the expression:

$$x = Ay^2 + By^4 + Cy^6 + Dy^8 + Ey^{10}$$

This has the effect of allowing the designer to follow the ellipsoid curve out to about a 40 mm diameter and then to choose values for the coefficients B, C, D and E so that the front surface curve flattens rapidly in the periphery. This is done in a continuous manner so that the lens no longer has the 'fried egg on a plate' appearance of a more traditional lenticular. This type of design is illustrated in Figure 8.12. The central zone A is an ellipsoid with the same characteristics as an aspheric lenticular having a diameter around 40 mm. The intermediate zone B has an ellipticotoroidal shape where the dramatic flattening occurs. The width of this zone is around 10 mm. The peripheral zone C is extended to give a total diameter around 70 mm.

8.9.2.3 Fitting distance sensitivity

The fitting distance is the distance from the lens back vertex to the centre of rotation of the eye. Aspheric lenses have a further advantage in that they are fairly insensitive to fitting distance changes. Table 8.5 shows the performance of the $+12.00$ D aspheric (ellipsoidal lenticular

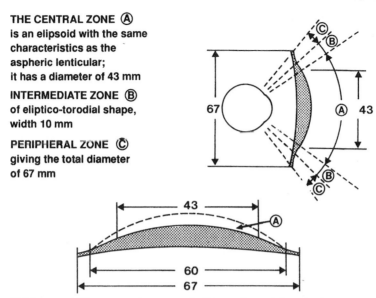

THE CENTRAL ZONE Ⓐ
is an elipsoid with the same
characteristics as the
aspheric lenticular;
it has a diameter of 43 mm

INTERMEDIATE ZONE Ⓑ
of eliptico-torodial shape,
width 10 mm

PERIPHERAL ZONE Ⓒ
giving the total diameter
of 67 mm

Thickness of 60 mm uncut compared with a polynomial aspheric

Figure 8.12. The shape of a polynomial convex aspherical surface. (Diagrams drawn from information provided by Essilor.)

TABLE 8.5 30° performance of the +12.00 D 40 mm diameter aspheric lenticular at different fitting distances

Fitting distance (mm)	F_t	F_s	MOP	OAE	MOE
23	+12.02	+11.54	+11.78	0.48	-0.22
25	+11.85	+11.49	+11.67	0.36	-0.33
27	+11.70	+11.45	+11.57	0.25	-0.43
29	+11.57	+11.41	+11.49	0.16	-0.51

F_t and F_s are the tangential and sagittal powers. This lens was designed for a fitting distance of 27 mm.

from Table 8.4) lenticular at a number of fitting distances. This is important because a lens of any given power will be fitted to patients with a variety of fitting distances and there is no way of measuring the fitting distance. Add to this the fact that patients may well end up wearing their spectacles on the end of their noses, then a lens design that is insensitive to fitting distance changes is desirable.

In comparison the spheric lenticular in Table 8.4 produces an OAE ranging from 0.93 to 1.35 D and an MOE ranging from +0.21 to +0.64 D. While the aspheric has a trade off between OAE and MOE as the fitting distance increases, the spheric simply gets worse in both

aspects and we can therefore regard the spheric design as being more sensitive to fitting distance changes and thus a less satisfactory design.

8.9.2.4 Transverse chromatic aberration (TCA) and rotatory distortion

TCA is the dispersion of white light in the tangential meridian. It is due to the prismatic effect away from the principal axis of the lens and results in tangential blur. If the prismatic effect at a point on the lens is P and the V value of the lens material is V then:

$$\text{TCA} = \frac{P}{V}$$

This equation shows why a high V value is desirable, since a high constringence produces low TCA. Strictly speaking the prismatic deviation in a thick lens must be derived by ray tracing which takes into account the lens surface powers and the lens thickness. However, the well used relationship

$$P = Fc$$

where F = lens power in dioptres and c = tangential distance to the optical centre of the lens in cm gives a good approximation for the prismatic deviation.

TABLE 8.6 TCA and distortion in aspheric and spheric forms of a +12.00 D lens for an ocular rotation of 30°

Lens	TCA(Δ)	Distortion (%)
Aspheric lenticular	0.35	8.24
Spheric lenticular	0.36	8.94
50 mm full aperture	0.37	9.18

Distortion is less with an aspheric lens because the tangential power is less than that in the spheric lens. This serves to reduce the deviation at the first surface. Table 8.6 compares the +12.00 D aspheric and spheric lenticulars from Table 8.4.   Although the differences are small, the aspheric has the lowest aberration values, which means that this design degrades and distorts the image less in oblique gaze than the other two best form designs. These effects can be reduced still further by keeping the vertex distance as small as possible; because a smaller ocular rotation is required for a given slope angle of the incident ray (see Figure 8.13).

8.9.3 Magnification

Although a patient using a pair of +1.00 D lenses for reading would count the 1% magnification as a bonus, the much larger magnification produced by an aphakic correction disturbs

spatial perception. Objects are perceived as being nearer in monocular vision with potential disturbance of stereopsis and binocular vision stability. For distant objects, the magnification of the retinal image is given by the relationship:

Spectacle magnification

$$= \text{power factor} \times \text{shape factor}$$

It will be recalled that the power factor $PF = 1/(1 - aF_v')$ where a is the distance from the lens back vertex to the entrance pupil of the eye. This equation shows that as distance a increases, the spectacle magnification will increase, therefore a small vertex distance is required to minimize the spectacle magnification and this is despite the fact that the lens BVP will have to be increased slightly to compensate for the decrease in vertex distance.

The shape factor $= 1/(1 - (t/n)F_1)$ where t is the lens central thickness and F_1 is its front surface power. This shows that the magnification is decreased by keeping the centre thickness small and the front surface power as low as possible. If we once again consider the lenses in Table 8.4 and assume a value of 13 mm for distance a we can draw up Table 8.7. Bearing in mind that a 1% magnification is noticeable, the smaller magnification of the aspheric lenticular is an evident improvement in performance.

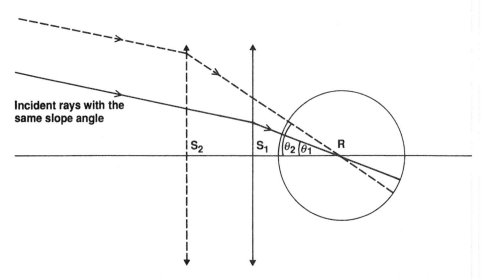

Figure 8.13. The greater fitting distance S_2R means that the eye must rotate through θ_2, the larger angle of rotation, when considering rays of the same slope angle. The eye is thus using a more peripheral region of the lens and this serves to increase the peripheral aberrations for any given lens design.

TABLE 8.7 Spectacle magnification with the full aperture and lenticular lenses of Table 8.4 ($a = 13$ mm)

Lens	Power factor	Shape factor	Magnification	Increase (%)
Full aperture	1.185	1.113	1.319	31.9
Spheric lenticular	1.185	1.091	1.293	29.3
Aspheric lenticular	1.185	1.072	1.270	27.0

8.9.4 Lack of accommodation

Stating the obvious, because the aphakic patient has lost her or his crystalline lens she or he requires help in focusing for near vision. The most important aspect to consider in prescribing and dispensing for the aphakic patient for near work is the near vision effectivity error (NVEE). Consider the following example in which the distance prescription is $+12.00$ D and the near vision spectacles determined using a refractor head or trial frame have a BVP of $+15.00$ D (see Figure 8.14). Assuming a plano-convex trial lens with the spherical surface towards the eye, then the reading lens will have a $+15.00$ D back surface power. The vergence leaving the lens must be $+12.00$ D for a clear retinal image to be maintained. If we assume that the trial lens is

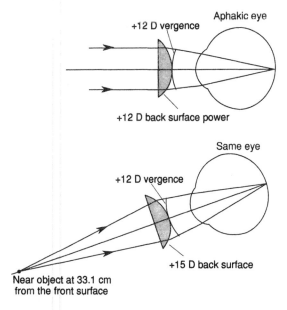

Near object at 33.1 cm from the front surface

Figure 8.14. Diagram used to discuss the near vision effectivity error (NVEE).

4 mm thick, paraxial calculation shows that the object will need to be positioned 33.1 cm from the lens front vertex. However, what happens if we order a $+15.00$ D prescription lens for close work? Firstly, manufacturers usually design their lenses for distance vision, so we take the best form for this power which is judged to be back surface power -2.00 D with an aspherical front surface (p value 0.65). We will assume that the centration and pantoscopic angle are correctly adjusted to make the lens' optical axis pass through the centre of rotation of the eye. If we assume that the eye's visual axis coincides with the lens' optical axis, the emergent vergence from the prescription lens for light from an object 33.1 cm from the lens front vertex is $+11.42$ D, which indicates that the lens is underpowered by 0.58 D when compared with the trial case lens. This is due to the fact that the NVEE is different in the two lens types, arising from using a trial lens with a plano front surface and a prescription lens with a high plus front surface with centre thickness differences between the two lenses. It is also likely that the wearer will use areas of the lens other than that of the optical centre. Figure 8.15 illustrates the situation and Table 8.8 lists the results of the calculations. The mean oblique image vergence (MOIV) is $(L_t' + L_s')/2$ where L_t' and L_s' are the emergent vergences in the tangential and sagittal planes measured at the vertex sphere.

Table 8.8 shows that the lens is underpowered along the axis and is increasingly underpowered as the eye rotates to use more peripheral parts of the lens. If the $+15.00$ D lens is ordered, the patient will be compelled to hold the object of interest further away in order to achieve the MOIV of $+12.00$ D. An oblique ray trace for the 10° rotation shows that the object must be held 7.4 cm further away than at the examination. This problem can be addressed by adding some extra positive power to the refraction result. Table 8.9 lists the extra power to be added to the refraction result. If, in our example above, we added $+0.50$ D to the BVP as suggested in Table 8.9, then the $+12.00$ D MOIV would be achieved with the object held at 35 cm. The error in the reading position is then only $35 - 33.1 = 1.9$ cm, which should be acceptable. The oblique NVEE remains almost the same as the fitting distance varies, so the recommendations above hold for the different fitting distances encountered with different patients.

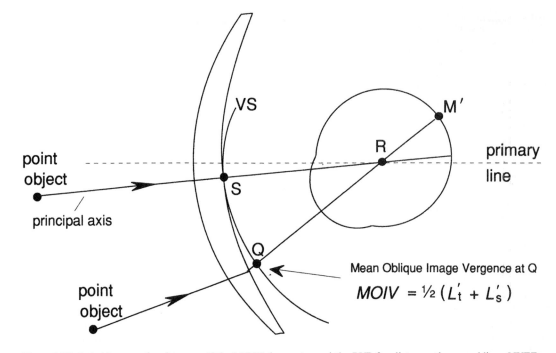

Figure 8.15. Aphakic correction for near. If the MOIV does not equal the BVP for distance, then an oblique NVEE exists.

TABLE 8.8 The near vision performance of a $+15.00$ D aspheric prescription lens

Ocular rotation (°)	Oblique astigmatism	MOIV	Expected vergence at VS	Vergence error at VS
0	$+0.00$	$+11.42$	$+12.00$	-0.58
5	$+0.00$	$+11.41$	$+12.00$	-0.59
10	$+0.00$	$+11.35$	$+12.00$	-0.65
15	$+0.01$	$+11.27$	$+12.00$	-0.73
20	$+0.03$	$+11.16$	$+12.00$	-0.84

MOIV = mean oblique image vergence. This is the mean of the tangential and the sagittal image vergences when oblique astigmatism is present. The tangential and sagittal image vergences will be the same when the oblique astigmatism is zero. VS is vertex sphere. All values listed are in dioptres.

TABLE 8.9 Extra positive power to be added to refraction result

Trial lens prescription for near vision	Correction for the stated addition		
	Add $+2.00$	Add $+2.50$	Add $+3.00$
$+8.00$	$+0.25$	$+0.25$	$+0.25$
$+8.50$	$+0.25$	$+0.25$	$+0.25$
$+9.00$	$+0.25$	$+0.25$	$+0.25$
$+9.50$	$+0.25$	$+0.25$	$+0.25$
$+10.00$	$+0.25$	$+0.25$	$+0.25$
$+10.50$	$+0.25$	$+0.25$	$+0.25$
$+11.00$	$+0.25$	$+0.25$	$+0.50$
$+11.50$	$+0.25$	$+0.25$	$+0.50$
$+12.00$	$+0.25$	$+0.25$	$+0.50$
$+12.50$	$+0.25$	$+0.50$	$+0.50$
$+13.00$	$+0.25$	$+0.50$	$+0.50$
$+13.50$	$+0.25$	$+0.50$	$+0.50$
$+14.00$	$+0.25$	$+0.50$	$+0.50$
$+14.50$	$+0.50$	$+0.50$	$+0.50$
$+15.00$	$+0.50$	$+0.50$	$+0.50$
$+15.50$	$+0.50$	$+0.50$	$+0.75$
$+16.00$	$+0.50$	$+0.50$	$+0.75$

This Table covers the central 10° zone. The values must be increased by around 50% for the 20° zone.
The Table is derived from a similar one published by Rodenstock.

8.9.4.1. Consequences of not compensating for NVEE

If NVEE is not compensated for, aphakic patients are compelled to hold reading material several centimetres further away than the optimum. In the majority of cases, the magnification allows an excellent acuity, often $\frac{6}{6}$ or better. So the patient would still be able to read N5 at a distance of 40 cm or more if the correction suggested above is omitted.

An additional factor to consider is that of depth of field. Assuming we have a 4 mm pupil, then the eye's depth of field closer than the focused position will be about 0.33 D. Since the required MOIV is $+12.00$ D for a clear retinal image, we can allow this to decrease to

$$12.00 - 0.33 = +11.67 \text{ D}$$

The object can be positioned 5 cm nearer the lens than when the depth of field is not considered.

There is yet another factor that may override our shortcomings. Suppose the + 15.00 D reading lens were to be moved deliberately or accidentally 5 mm further from the eye. If we then assume that the optical centre is 2 mm lower, so the wearer looks very nearly along the optical axis of the lens, the vergence at the eye will turn out exactly right, an initial vertex distance of 13 mm having been assumed. So the question arises as to whether or not aphakes fiddle with their glasses until a better focus is achieved in a spectacle correction that has not been compensated for NVEE. Nevertheless, optometrists should strive to maintain the highest levels of precision and to this end, Table 8.9 should be consulted when considering the near prescription of an aphakic patient.

8.9.5 Field of view

There are two points to consider:

(a) The field of view at the limit of the lens aperture.
(b) Making the right and left fields of view coincide through the segments of bifocals in patients with binocular vision.

8.9.5.1 The field of fixation

Figure 8.16(a) illustrates the constriction of the static visual field of view. Figure 8.16(b) illustrates the constriction of the dynamic field (field of fixation). Both of these are produced by the prismatic effect of the high plus lens which inevitably produces a ring scotoma.

Figure 8.17 illustrates the phenomenon called the 'Jack in the box effect'. The object A is seen in the periphery by the eye in the primary position Figure 8.17(a). The eye then turns to look at the object, and the lateral movement of the pupil results in the limiting light ray imposing a further constriction of the field, so that object A is now covered by the change in position of the ring scotoma Figure 8.17(b). This means that the object of interest disappears as the wearer looks towards it, only to reappear when the eye returns to the primary position. This phenomenon may not be as distressing as is sometimes suggested because people tend to turn their heads to look at objects in the periphery. It must be noted that rotating the eye about 30° from the primary position in order to look through the lens periphery is not particularly comfortable.

The polynomial design, already described, provides us with a lens where the prismatic effect increases as we move away from the optical centre to the limit of the ellipsoidal zone and after this the prism decreases as we move to more eccentric positions. This means that there

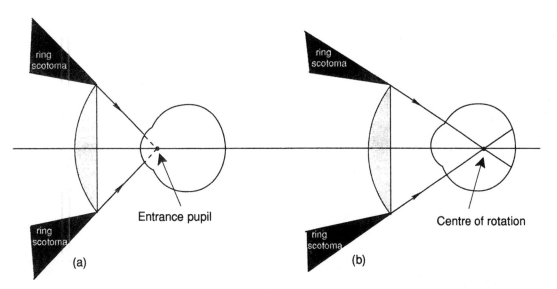

Figure 8.16. The ring scotoma (a) for the static field of view and (b) for the field of fixation.

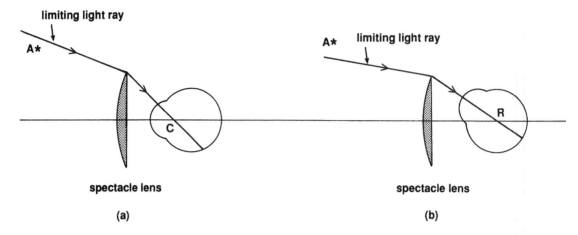

Figure 8.17.(a) The limiting light ray passes through the centre of curvature of the refracting surface (C). Thus the object A is within the field of vision. (b) The limiting ray now passes through the centre of rotation of the eye (R) and object A disappears into the ring scotoma.

is little or no prism at the lens periphery and consequently there is little or no ring scotoma (see Figure 8.18). In a 40 mm diameter +12.00 D aspheric lenticular (not a polynomial), the deviation of a ray at 35° of ocular rotation is a little less than 14°. This is the angular size of the ring scotoma for the field of fixation. At 50 m distance, an object 12.5 m wide is occluded by the scotoma. Fitting the lens as close as possible to the eye will help with the problem. As a practical analogy, think about walking closer to a window – your field of view increases and the window surround is less obtrusive.

8.9.5.2 Bifocal inset

The problem with bifocal inset involves making the eyes look through the centres of the segments when fixing on a point on the median line at the requisite working distance. When this is achieved the two fields of view will coincide.

Figure 8.19 illustrates the path of the chief ray passing through the centre of the segment and the eye's centre of rotation. The inset of the bifocal is the horizontal distance OQ which will ensure that the right and left fields of view for near vision will coincide. The inset OQ is derived as follows:

bifocal inset $= s \tan \theta$

Using paraxial optics for refraction at the lens, the image point is taken to be a distance h' from

(a)

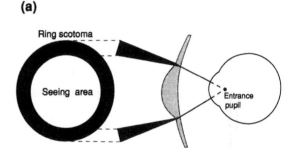

Ring scotoma in a classic lenticular with a visible demarcation between the central optic zone and the margin of the lens

(b)

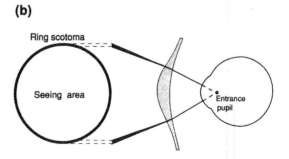

Much reduced ring scotoma with a polynomial aspheric lens

Figure 8.18. Comparison of the non-seeing area (ring scotoma) in lenticular and polynomial aspheric lenses. (a) A pronounced ring scotoma in a classic lenticular lens. (b) The much reduced width of the scotoma with a polynomial aspheric lens.

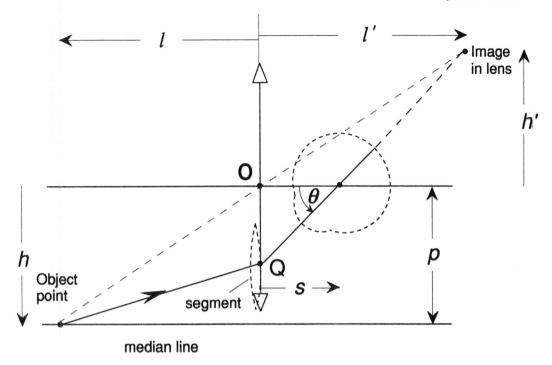

Figure 8.19. Determination of the bifocal inset to make the reading portion fields coincide. θ = eye rotation; p = semi-pupillary distance; OQ = inset.

the optical axis of the lens and the object point a distance h ($= p$) from the axis. Then, from the magnification expression,

$$h' = h(L/L') = p(L/L')$$

and

$$\tan \theta = \frac{h'}{l' - s}$$

$$= \frac{p(L/L')}{l' - s}$$

$$= \frac{pL}{1 - sL'}$$

We can now substitute for $\tan \theta$ into the expression for bifocal inset and obtain

$$\text{bifocal inset} = \frac{spL}{1 - sL'}$$

Writing $s = 1/S$ and $L' = L + F$ and substituting for s and L' in the last expression, we have

$$\frac{(1/S)pL}{1 - (1/S)(L + F)}$$

Multiplying this by S/S leaves us with

$$\frac{pL}{S - (L + F)}$$

Thus

$$\text{bifocal inset} = p[L/(L + F - S)]$$

where p is the semi-pupillary distance (semi-PD) measured for each eye (mm), L is the object vergence (D), F is the power of the distance correction (D) and S is $1/s$ where s is the fitting distance assumed to be 0.025 m.

Thus $S = 1/0.025 = 40$ D.

Table 8.10 lists typical inset values. It illustrates that the all too frequent practice of asking for a 2 mm inset of the segments is completely inadequate in the case of the aphakic patient.

8.9.6 Centration and prisms

In the UK it is likely that, in the absence of any instructions from the optometrist, the lens will be glazed with its optical centre on the horizontal centre line (datum line), some 5 to 6 mm below the centre of the pupil in the primary

TABLE 8.10 Bifocal inset as a function of object distance, semi-PD and distance prescription (to the nearest $\frac{1}{2}$ mm)

Semi-PD (mm)	Distance Rx (D)	Working distance (cm)			
		25	33	40	50
30	+10.00	4.0	3.0	2.5	2.5
	+12.00	4.0	3.0	2.5	2.5
	+14.00	4.5	3.5	3.0	2.5
	+16.00	5.0	4.0	3.0	2.5
32.5	+10.00	4.0	3.0	3.0	2.5
	+12.00	4.5	3.5	3.0	2.5
	+14.00	5.0	4.0	3.0	2.5
	+16.00	5.0	4.0	3.5	3.0
35	+10.00	4.5	3.5	3.0	2.5
	+12.00	5.0	4.0	3.0	2.5
	+14.00	5.0	4.0	3.5	3.0
	+16.00	5.5	4.5	4.0	3.0

position of gaze. It is assumed that the lens' optical axis will pass through the eye's centre of rotation, because this is a necessary lens design criterion to preserve the design performance. This is achieved by adjusting the angle of side to alter the pantoscopic tilt, as in Figure 8.20.

It is easy to derive the approximation, called the dispenser's rule, that for each 1 mm lowering of the optical centre the pantoscopic angle should be increased by 2°. Horizontal positioning of the optical centres depends on the semi-PDs. It is not acceptable to assume equal semi-PDs with the lens power required for the aphake because the subsequent failure of the principal axis to pass through the centre of rotation of the eye will degrade the image to that determined by the off-axis performance of the lens. Similarly, bowing the frame to follow the head contours has the same effect of deviating the optical axis away from the centre of rotation. Bowing is done to increase the lateral field of view but this is better maximized by fitting the lenses as close to the eyes as possible which will provide a more than adequate field with the large-diameter lenses currently available. High-powered plus lenses centred for distance vision increase the amount of convergence required for near vision. This has already been illustrated in Figure 8.19 where the ocular rotation θ can be determined instead of the segment inset from the relationship:

$$\tan \theta = \frac{\text{inset}}{\text{fitting distance}} = \frac{OQ}{s}$$

The amount of convergence required for fixation at 35 cm from the spectacle plane is given for various semi-PDs in Table 8.11 which

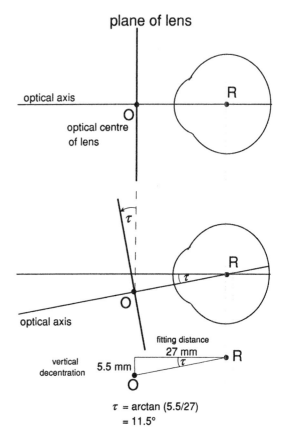

$$\tau = \arctan (5.5/27)$$
$$= 11.5°$$

Figure 8.20. For each millimetre decentration down from the primary line, the pantoscopic tilt τ should be increased by 2°.

TABLE 8.11 Convergence in prism dioptres (Δ) required when fixing an object point at 35 cm from the spectacle plane on the median line for various semi-PDs, fitting distances and distance prescriptions. Cornea to centre of rotation assumed constant at 14 mm

Distance Rx (D)	Fitting distance (mm)	Semi-PD		
		30 (mm)	32.5 (mm)	35 (mm)
+0.00	23	8.0	8.7	9.4
	25	8.0	8.7	9.3
	27	8.0	8.6	9.3
+10.00	23	10.3	11.1	12.0
	25	10.4	11.3	12.2
	27	10.6	11.5	12.4
+12.00	23	10.8	11.8	12.7
	25	11.1	12.0	13.0
	27	11.4	12.3	13.3
+14.00	23	11.5	12.5	13.5
	25	11.9	12.9	13.9
	27	12.3	13.3	14.3

includes the emmetropic case for comparison. From the results we see that convergence will be slightly less for a closer fitting lens.

The high power of the lenses means that a substantial prism can be induced by modest decentration. However, if the lens has an aspherical surface, it should not be decentred to produce a prismatic effect for a prescribed prism. The prism must be worked into the lens (by grinding the two surfaces at an angle) in order to keep the vertex of the aspherical surface in the correct position in front of the pupil centre.

8.9.7 Protection from ultraviolet (UV) radiation

The crystalline lens normally absorbs the UVA radiation (315–390 nm) but in the aphakic eye UVA can penetrate to the retina. There is now strong evidence that this may cause retinal damage and should therefore be removed by prescribing a UV-absorbing tint.

8.9.8 Dispensing spectacles for the aphakic – Summary

(a) Frames.
  (i) Should be lightweight with thin rims to minimize any ring scotoma.
  (ii) Should possess large adjustable pads, if possible, to allow some vertical movement of the optical centres to correspond to the pantoscopic tilt and allow minimum vertex distance fitting. It may, however, be necessary to consider a regular bridge in order to spread the weight of the spectacles over a large area.
  (iii) Should have a distance between centres (boxing system) as close as possible to the patient's pupillary distance, because this centres the lenses in the frame. Excessively upswept shapes should be avoided since shaping the lens will cut into the thicker central portion.

(b) Minimum vertex distance ensures
  (i) a maximum field of view;
  (ii) a minimum convergence demand;
  (iii) a minimum retinal image size;
  (iv) a minimum size for the image of the wearer's eyes;
  (v) minimal effects from the peripheral aberrations of the correcting lens.

(c) Centration
  (i) Accurate centring is necessary not only to prevent differential prismatic effects but to centre the vertex of an aspherical surface. Accurate centration also ensures the best oblique gaze performance with both aspheric and spheric lenses. For distance correction, the semi-PDs should be recorded and the lenses centred accordingly, even in the case of the unilateral aphake.
  (ii) Near-vision lenses should be centred according to the semi-NCDs (near centration distances), which must be measured. This minimizes the induced prism but the lens optical axis will not run through the centres of rotation of the eyes in the horizontal plane. This could only be achieved by bowing the frame so that the lenses are angled into a converged configuration which would look cosmetically odd.
  (iii) Bifocal segments must be inset to make the right and left reading portion fields of view coincide.

(d) NVEE should be compensated.
(e) A UV-absorbing tint should be incorporated into the lens.

Recommended reading

Bennett, A.G. and Rabbetts, R.B. *Clinical Visual Optics*, 2nd edn, Butterworths, London (1989)

Jalie, M. *The Principles of Ophthalmic Lenses*, 3rd edn, Association of Dispensing Opticians, London (1977)

Tunnacliffe, A.H. *Introduction to Visual Optics*, Association of Dispensing Opticians, London (1984)

Contact lens correction

William A. Douthwaite

9.1 Contact lenses in the ageing eye

The aphakic eye is likely to belong to an elderly patient and this has a number of implications for the contact lens practitioner. The basal metabolic rate will be lower and the absence of the crystalline lens produces a higher oxygen partial pressure in the aqueous at the endothelium. However, the decrease in lid tension along with the possibility of ptosis, ectropion and incomplete blinking may produce fitting difficulties, as will the reduction in tear volume. Where the surgery has involved a scleral or corneal section, the overall sensitivity of the cornea to pain will be reduced which means that an important protective mechanism of the anterior eye has been rendered less effective. Also, surgical intervention may result in the induction of an astigmatic component in the cornea around 1.00 to 3.00 D. There is also likely to be endothelial cell loss along with the possibility of macular oedema, retinal detachment and opacification of the lens capsule. Any of these latter sequelae may influence the final visual acuity attained. One final point to be made is that removal of the crystalline lens, which is opaque to light wavelengths below 375 nm in the elderly (310 nm in the young), results in light with a wavelength down to 290 nm reaching the retina. There is an increasing body of evidence to suggest that light of this short wavelength will damage the retinal cells. Therefore any type of optical correction should incorporate a suitable ultraviolet filter [1].

9.2 Astigmatism

The problems of corneal astigmatism can be dealt with effectively by using a rigid spherical corneal lens or a toric corneal or soft lens. If the practitioner wishes to avoid using a toric soft lens, then a spherical soft lens could be used in conjunction with a spectacle correction which incorporates the astigmatic element. It may well be worth considering a bifocal correction here, where the distance section corrects the astigmatism and the reading addition provides the extra positive spherical power required for near work.

9.3 Stabilization time after surgery

If a practitioner intends to correct an aphakic patient with contact lenses, it is advisable to allow some time for the postsurgical refraction to stabilize. The time interval recommended appears to vary from 3 weeks to 6 months, depending on the authority consulted. This is obviously an unsatisfactory guide and in any case it may be preferable to rely more on the stability of measurements like keratometry and refraction. Mandell [2] suggests taking refraction and keratometry readings on a weekly basis and waiting until the refraction, the corneal radius of curvature and principal meridian orientation results are stable over a 3-week period, before instituting the fitting. Before fitting commences, an ophthalmological opinion must be sought, the eye should not be inflamed, and the incision should be quiet and healed with no corneal staining or dry spots. A longer waiting period may be appropriate when lens handling by the patient is poor so as to avoid any untoward trauma to a very recently healed eye.

The keratometric measurements should not present any problems. The astigmatism measured by the keratometer will give an indication of the astigmatic correction required, although this may be misleading if the pupil is not central. The mire images may show some distortion and the principal meridians may not be mutually perpendicular which means a one-position instrument may give inappropriate results. If a practitioner uses such an instrument, it would be better operated as though it were a two-position instrument.

9.4 The influence of cataract surgery

The type of contact lens fitted, the time of fitting and the possible complications arising during aftercare checks may be influenced by the surgical procedure adopted.

9.4.1 Intracapsular extraction

In this technique, an incision is made from 9 to 3 o'clock around the superior limbus. A peripheral iridectomy is usually performed to prevent iris prolapse and pupillary block. A round pupil is usually preserved. Occasionally, a whole sector of the iris is removed leaving a keyhole pupil. If the patient has a low upper lid, then this will cover most of the absent iris and the contact lens fitting can proceed as for a normal pupil. A high positioned upper lid, however, may result in significant visual disturbance when a corneal contact lens is used. In these cases, a scleral or a soft contact lens may give a better visual result. In fact, any procedure which results in a decentred pupil, will point the contact lens practitioner in the direction of the soft and scleral lenses. The type of suture employed at the end of the operation and the tension applied will affect the corneal shape.

Astigmatism may be induced which, if large, can complicate the contact lens fitting.

Possible complications arising from the surgery are as follows:

(a) Vitreous prolapse. If this occurs, it must be attended to within a few days to prevent corneal damage and severe oedema.
(b) Corneal striae. These may be apparent, indicating a significant amount of oedema.
(c) Endothelial trauma. This will be accompanied by oedema and will display polymegathism/pleomorphism, if a slit-lamp with sufficient magnification is available. Bullous keratopathy may develop in severe cases causing pain and loss of vision.
(d) Incomplete incision closure. This may result in a leak developing which may lead to a shallow anterior angle. Alternatively, epithelial cells may grow through the incision into the anterior chamber.
(e) Iris prolapse. This again arises from inadequate suturing or postsurgical trauma. It may lead to peripheral anterior synechiae and glaucoma.
(f) Infection. Bacterial infection will become apparent soon after surgery but fungal infection may not be apparent for several weeks.

9.4.2 Extracapsular extraction

A smaller incision is required at the limbus with this approach. The lack of trauma, rapid recovery, little change in corneal curvature and fewer postoperative complications give this technique some obvious advantages, not the least of which is that a contact lens fitting can be initiated earlier than with the intracapsular technique, which may be typically 3–4 months after the operation.

9.5 Contact lens correction of the monocular aphake

The most striking improvement to be gained in transferring from a spectacle to a contact lens correction occurs in the unilateral aphake. This is due to the reduced magnification produced by the contact lens correction. The factors that determine spectacle magnification (the power factor and the shape factor) can be applied to a contact lens correction. It will be observed that an eye which was close to being emmetropic before lens removal will undergo an increase in retinal image size of around 30% when corrected by spectacles (see Secion 8.7). This increase is reduced to less than 10% with a contact lens correction. Reference to the power factor and shape factor equations illustrates that this is due to the much reduced distance between the contact lens and the entrance pupil of the eye and the fact that the contact lens is much thinner than the equivalent spectacle lens (see Sections 8.8.1 and 8.8.2).

There is no possibility of fusing the two retinal images into a single binocular image when the unilateral aphake is corrected by spectacles. The low magnification with a contact lens correction is small enough to allow fusion of the images from the aphakic and non-aphakic eyes. It should, however, be noted that some patients are disturbed by image size differences as small as 1% and therefore binocular vision difficulties may still arise. Guillon and Warland [3] found that, in their study, most of the unilateral aphakic patients wearing a contact lens achieved only 140 s of arc on the Titmus stereotest, and 80% displayed intermittent suppression.

Osamu *et al.* [4] measured the aniseikonia in patients using intraocular lenses (IOLs), contact lenses and spectacles and found aniseikonia of 2.8%, 4.6% and 17.8% respectively. The respective group values for good stereo acuity were 68.4%, 40.7% and 0%. More binocular vision difficulties may be experienced if the aphakic eye is the non-dominant eye.

If the monocular aphakic patient requires a spectacle correction for the phakic eye, a contact lens could be prescribed for the aphakic eye with too much positive power. This extra power is then neutralized by a negative spectacle lens positioned at an above-average vertex distance. This will minify the retinal image and consequently reduce the disparity in the retinal image sizes of the two eyes.

9.5.1 Calculation of spectacle magnification

Let us consider an emmetropic patient who has a cataract removed from the right eye and is subsequently fitted with a corneal contact lens with a Back Optic Zone Radius (BOZR) of 7.80 mm which gives an alignment fit. It is fair to assume that the alignment fit produces a thin afocal fluid lens which will not affect the size of the retinal image. The contact lens will typically require a back vertex power (BVP) of $+12.00$ D to correct the eye for distance vision. If we decide to overcorrect the eye by $+5.00$ D, then the BVP becomes $+17.00$ D. If we assume a contact lens central thickness of 0.6 mm with the entrance pupil 3 mm behind the anterior cornea and a contact lens refractive index of 1.490, then we can calculate the spectacle magnification. We first need to know the front surface power of the contact lens and this can be calculated using the step-along method (see Figure 9.1).

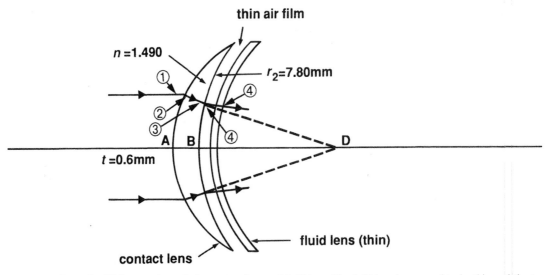

Figure 9.1 The path of light rays through the contact lens and fluid lens. The fluid lens is assumed to be thin and the two lenses are separated by a thin air film. The light rays are assumed to be paraxial. The numbers within the circles identify the vergences.

The contact lens back surface power F_2 is

$$\frac{-490}{7.8} = -62.82 \text{ D}$$

Vergence (D)	Distance (mm)
④ = +17.00	
F_2 = −62.82 (subtract)	

$$③ = +79.82 \rightarrow \frac{1000}{79.82} \rightarrow 12.53 = \text{BD}$$
$$00.4 \text{ (add) } t/n$$

$$② = +77.35 \leftarrow \frac{1000}{12.93} \leftarrow 12.93 = \text{AD}$$

① = +00.00   (subtract)

F_1 = +77.35

The spectacle magnification due to the contact lens is now calculated using:

$$\text{Power factor} = \frac{1}{1 - aF_v'} \quad \text{(see Section 8.8.1)}$$

and

$$\text{Shape factor} = \frac{1}{1 - (t/n)F_1} \quad \text{(see Section 8.8.2)}$$

where

Spectacle magnification

$$= \text{power factor} \times \text{shape factor}$$

F_v' is the BVP (D) of the correcting lens, a is the distance from the back vertex of the lens to the entrance pupil of the eye in metres, F_1 is the front surface power (D) of the correcting lens and t/n is the reduced thickness of the correcting lens in metres.

$$\text{Power factor} = \frac{1}{1 - (0.003 \times 17)} = 1.0537$$

$$\text{Shape factor} = \frac{1}{1 - (0.0004 \times 77.35)} = 1.0319$$

Spectacle
magnification = 1.0537 × 1.0319 = 1.0873

Thus the image is 8.73% larger than the image in the uncorrected eye.

If the contact lens was fitted steep, the fluid lens would have to be considered in the same way, and the spectacle magnification of the fluid lens would need to be multiplied by that of the contact lens in order to arrive at the total spectacle magnification. Thus, a steep fit would serve to increase the magnification of the retinal image.

The question now arises as to what retinal image minification can be achieved when a −5.50 D spectacle lens is used to neutralize the excess +5.00 D power of the contact lens. A −5.50 D spectacle lens will have an effective power of −5.00 D at the cornea for a vertex distance of 15 mm.

A typical spectacle lens made from Crown glass will have a front surface power of +3.50 D and a centre thickness of 1.5 mm. The shape factor of this lens produces a magnification around 0.3%, therefore the shape factor can be ignored.

The power factor for a vertex distance (lens to cornea) of 15 mm is: $1/[1 - 0.018 \times -5.5)]$ = 0.91. Thus the retinal image is reduced in size by 9%.

If the contact lens was over plussed by 3.00 D, the spectacle magnification would be 8% and the −3.00 D spectacle lens at 15 mm would minify the image by 5%.

A convenient approximation to deduce the spectacle lens required for the chosen vertex distance is arrived at by regarding the contact lens–spectacle lens system as a Galilean (minifying) telescope.

The initial procedure is to determine the spectacle magnification due to the contact lens (with no overcorrection) by determining the power and shape factors of the contact and fluid lenses and multiplying these together. A reversed Galilean telescope is then required to minify the image by the same amount.

Figure 9.2 illustrates a Galilean telescope set for distance:

$$\text{Magnification} = \frac{\text{Power of eyepiece}}{\text{Power of objective}}$$

$$= \frac{F_e}{F_o} = \frac{f_o}{f_e}$$

where f_o is the focal length of the objective and f_e is the focal length of the eyepiece. Also $f_e = f_o - s$ where s is the separation between the objective and the eyepiece.

$$\text{Magnification } m = \frac{f_o}{f_o - s}$$

$$= \frac{1}{1 - (s/f_o)}$$

$$= \frac{1}{1 - sF_o}$$

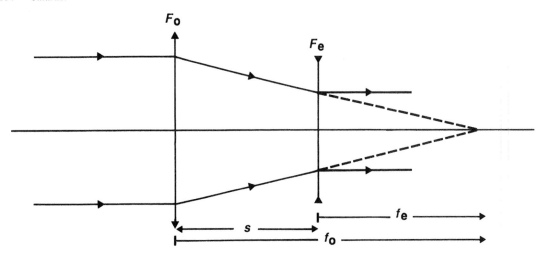

Figure 9.2 The Galilean telescope. F_o is the power of the objective; F_e is the power of the eyepiece; f_o is the focal length of the objective; f_e is the focal length of the eyepiece; s is the separation between the objective and the eyepiece.

Therefore

$$1 - sF_o = 1/m$$

$$sF_o = 1 - (1/m)$$

$$F_o = [1 - (1/m)]/s$$

Let us now take an example. The aphakic eye is corrected by an alignment-fitting contact lens of **BOZR** 7.80 mm, central thickness 0.6 mm, **BVP** +12.00 D and is made of polymethylmethacrylate (PMMA) (refractive index 1.490).

The power of the back surface

$$F_2 = \frac{-490}{7.8} = -62.82 \text{ D}$$

Figure 9.1 shows the path of the light rays through this lens, and the step-along method can be used to determine the front surface power F_1.

	Vergence (D)	Distance (mm)
④ =	+12.00	
F_2 =	−62.82	(subtract)

$$③ = +74.82 \rightarrow \frac{1000}{74.82} \rightarrow 13.37 = \text{BD}$$
$$00.4 \quad \text{(add)} \; t/n$$

$$② = +72.62 \leftarrow \frac{1000}{13.77} \leftarrow 13.77 = \text{AD}$$

① =	+00.00	(subtract)

$$F_1 = +72.62$$

Power factor $= 1/[(1 - (0.003 \times 12)] = 1.0373$

Shape factor $= 1/[(1 - (0.0004 \times 72.62)]$
$$= 1.0299$$

Spectacle magnification $= 1.0373 \times 1.0299$
$$= 1.0683$$

Thus the contact lens is increasing the retinal image size by 6.83% and we require a reversed telescope to minify the image by the same amount. Thus, the magnification required is 0.9317 times (approximately 93.2%).

We can now substitute our numbers into the telescope equations assuming a vertex distance of 15 mm:

$$F_o = [1 - (1/m)]/s$$
$$F_o = [1 - (1/0.9317)]/0.015$$
$$= -4.89 \text{ D}$$

Thus, we need a -5.00 D spectacle lens at 15 mm vertex distance which will have an effective power at the contact lens (found by using the step-along method as described in Section 8.4) of -4.65 D. Therefore, the contact lens will be overplussed by 4.75 D to give a BVP of $+16.75$ D.

If we decided to go for a back vertex distance of 12 mm in the above example, the telescope equation would be:

$$F_o = [1 - (1/0.9317)]/0.012$$
$$= -6.11 \text{ D}$$

So it is easy to deduce the spectacle lens power required for any back vertex distance.

The shape factor equation illustrates the fact that the retinal image size is dependent on the central thickness of the contact lens and the fluid lens. The most appropriate contact lens for the monocular aphakic must, therefore, be as thin as possible and fitted to avoid a steep fit in order to keep the image size as small as possible. If binocular vision problems persist, an opaque contact lens may be used as an occluder on the eye with the poorer visual acuity (see Figure 9.3).

9.5.2 Relative vertical prism

Any spectacle correction where there is a significant difference between the power of the right and left lens will produce a relative prism when the eyes use regions of the lenses other than that immediately surrounding the lens optical centre. Assume that the spectacle lenses are centred for distance work and the near visual point (NVP) is 10 mm below and 2 mm in from the optical centre of each lens. If we apply the relationship:

$$P = Fc$$

where P is the prismatic deviation in prism dioptres (Δ), F is the power of the correcting spectacle lens (D) and c is the distance from the optical centre to the point on the lens through which the visual axis passes (cm), we can calculate the prismatic effect of each lens.

The horizontal prism will be small because of the small distance c (0.2 mm), and the eyes can cope with any relative prism by simply converging more for positive lenses and less for negative lenses. However, there are only limited fusional reserves in the vertical meridian. If a patient is wearing a +2.00 D lens before the right eye, then the vertical prism at the NVP will be

$2 \times 1 = 2\Delta$ base up.

If the left eye requires a +12.00 D lens, then the prism at the NVP will be

$12 \times 1 = 12\Delta$ base up.

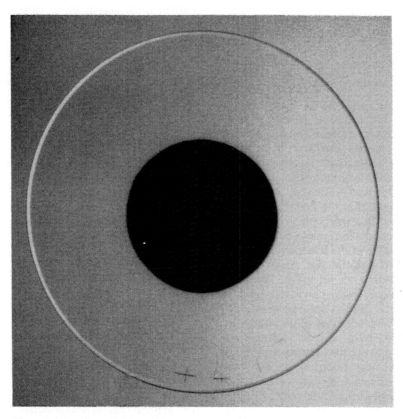

Figure 9.3 A soft contact lens with an opaque pupil.

Thus the relative vertical prism will be 10Δ base up left eye and this will produce vertical diplopia.

This example illustrates the notion that we can deduce the relative vertical prism in the clinical situation by multiplying the right–left lens power difference by the distance from the optical centre to the point of concern. The base will be up in the more hyperopic eye and down in the more myopic eye, when the visual axes are depressed. A contact lens correction will result in the correcting lens moving with the eye when it rotates to depress the visual axis. Thus, the decentration distance c remains at or close to 0 and no significant vertical prism is induced.

9.6 Contact lens correction of the bilateral aphake

A contact lens correction results in a more normal image size with a reduction in peripheral aberrations, owing to the fact that the contact lens moves with the eye and this means that there are distinct advantages for the bilateral aphake, not the least of which is that the static and dynamic fields of view are normal (see Section 8.9.5).

9.6.1 Correction for near vision

The fact that the aphake is incapable of accommodation has led some practitioners to suggest the addition of some extra positive power to the distance correction, in order to help the aphakic patient with intermediate and close work. However, caution on the part of the enthusiastic optometrist is advised. Douthwaite *et al.* [5] have noted that the positive spherical aberration present in a high plus contact lens produces a correction which may well be around 2.00 D more positive in the lens periphery than at its centre. Thus, an aphakic patient whose contact lenses ride high when the eyes are depressed for close work may well manage without the extra positive power mentioned above. If a reading addition is required, this could be provided by a pair of reading spectacles which simply contain the reading addition. Often, the near addition is less than expected. This reduced addition can be attributed to the removal of the finite vertex distance present in a powerful distance spectacle correction, which results in a decrease in the ocular

accommodation required to view near objects when positive power contact lenses are worn by the hyperope. A decrease in the power of the reading addition is likely in the case of the aphakic, where the ocular accommodation is replaced by the reading addition, remembering that the vertex distance will have no significant effect on the power of the addition if it is less than 4.00 D.

9.6.2 The over refraction

If the eye was nearly emmetropic before surgery, a contact lens power around +12.00 D will be required. It is advisable to have trial lenses of suitable power. This will ensure that the lens in the refractor head or trial frame during the over refraction will be of low power and this means that the vertex distance is of little or no consequence. Also, there is less possibility of inducing the errors that can arise when a contact lens of inappropriate power is used for the over refraction. A +12.00 D contact lens will mimic more accurately the behaviour of the lens ultimately ordered. Even so, the aphakic patient must accept more variability in visual acuity and refractive error than occurs in a typical ametrope.

In the case of a soft lens wearer, the over refraction may produce an unexpected result, partly because of the lens flexure (see Figure 9.4), which has been fully described by Bennett [6]. The power change in the soft contact lens is given by:

$$\Delta F_v' = -300t(1/r_2'^2 - 1/2r_2^2)$$

where $\Delta F_v'$ is the change in the BVP, t is the centre thickness, r_2 is the original back surface radius and r_2' is the new back surface radius after flexure.

This equation shows the following.

(a) The change in power is independent of the BVP of the contact lens.
(b) The BVP will become more negative as the curves steepen.
(c) The power change will be greater in thicker lenses.

It is inevitable that the centre thickness of a high plus lens will be substantial.

9.7 Contact lens selection

The general type of lens selected will depend on personal circumstances. Rigid corneal lenses are

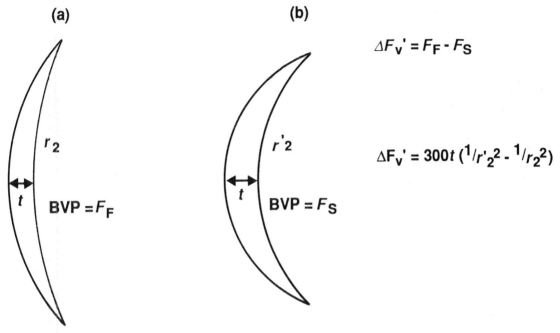

(a)

r_2

t

BVP $= F_F$

(b)

$\Delta F_v{'} = F_F - F_S$

r'_2

t

BVP $= F_S$

$$\Delta F_v{'} = 300t \left(\frac{1}{r'_2{}^2} - \frac{1}{r_2{}^2}\right)$$

Figure 9.4 The change in BVP induced when the soft contact lens (a) flexes into a steeper curved form (b).

more robust than their soft counterpart and may be a safer proposition where hygiene compliance is poor. The rigid spherical lens will also fully correct the corneal astigmatism. This correction is provided by the fluid lens which possesses a spherical front and toroidal back surface. The toroidal back surface corrects 90% of the anterior surface corneal astigmatism (derived from the ratio of the refractivities of the tears and the cornea), and the posterior corneal surface neutralizes the remaining 10%.

It is worth considering a gas-permeable material, particularly where a large diameter lens is required, to provide adequate pupillary cover. Any pupil–iris abnormalities arising from the surgery will require special consideration in this respect. It is, however, worth noting the generalization that, as the permeability of the gas-permeable lens material increases, there is an increased tendency for the lens to flex on the eye and thereby transmit an astigmatic error. The considerable centre thickness required for the high plus power will improve the resistance to flexure. The high-permeability materials offer the possibility of an extended-wear regime but the large central thickness will limit oxygen transmission through the lens. It must be noted here that the aphakic eye may have a lower atmospheric oxygen demand than the non-

aphakic eye, therefore extended wear with a gas-permeable lens is a possibility. However, the use of PMMA with all its attendant advantages should not be ruled out for daily wear.

If a rigid corneal lens is uncomfortable, then the soft lens must be considered. This general type may be particularly useful where the pupil is eccentric, or there is a peripheral iridectomy. The soft lens also offers the option of extended wear.

9.8 Corneal lenses

In general, the normal fitting criteria can be applied to the aphakic eye. The diameters employed in the aphake tend to be around 0.5 mm larger than those used for more routine refractive errors. The larger diameter is required to assist in stabilizing movement and improving centration.

Centration is a particular problem arising from the fact that the high positive power of the contact lens encourages the lens to ride low, with little promise of support from the lower lid, because of the weak lid tension found in the elderly patient. This, coupled with a decentred pupil or iridectomy, can produce a poor visual performance. Ideally, a fitting set made up with aphakic powers should be used in order to observe and assess lens centration and movement most effectively. The large diameters and the high positive power will produce thick and heavy lenses unless a lenticulated design is used.

A typical trial set might therefore consist of lenses with:

- BOZR from 7.00 to 8.00 mm in 0.1 mm steps
- Back Optic Zone Diameter (BOZD) of 7.50 mm
- Back Peripheral Radius (BPR) equal to the BOZR +0.6 mm
- Total Diameter (TD) of 9.80 mm
- Front Optic Zone Diameter (FOZD) of 7.60 mm with junction thickness around 0.14 mm
- Edge thickness 0.25 mm

The increase in lens thickness from the lenticular junction to the edge produces what is described as a negative carrier (see Figure 9.5). The intention is to trap the carrier under the upper lid, resulting in the lens riding in a higher and, hopefully, better centred position. When assessing the fit, the pupil should be contained within the area of the back optic zone. If this is

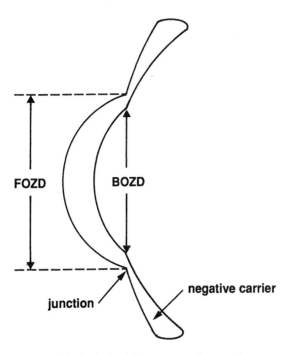

FOZD   **BOZD**

negative carrier

junction

Figure 9.5 The lenticulated bicurve corneal contact lens with a negative carrier.

not achieved, then image flare and diplopia may be experienced by the patient. Improved centration may be achieved by using shorter back surface radii (steepening the fit), although this may compromise the physiological compatibility of the lens.

Occasionally, a very small corneal lens may prove effective, but this will only work when the lens centres well and the eye has a well-centred pupil. The total diameter could be as small as 7.00 mm with a BOZD of 6.50 mm and a flat peripheral radius around 12.50 mm. This approach can be considered in cases prone to corneal fragility and oedema. These lenses work better on steep rather than flat corneas. The centre thickness of this type of lens will be around 0.3 to 0.4 mm in typical aphakic powers. However, this very small lens is going to produce definite handling problems for the aphakic wearer.

Aspheric back surface lenses can be fitted by following the general fitting recommendations. Some practitioners claim that the centration is improved when compared with the equivalent multicurve lens. Aspheric front surfaces could be used to correct the aberrations which arise in high positive power lenses with steep surface curves, and a better visual acuity may ensue. Calculations reveal that the aspheric back surface lens can possess an average thickness which is less than that of an equivalent multicurve, even when the central thickness is the same. This only occurs when the aspheric surface has a much lower p value than that currently used by lens manufacturers. It must also be remembered that aspheric surfaces are astigmatic outside the apical region and, in consequence, any lens which is decentred in relation to the pupil centre will display a reduced optical performance. If the corneal toricity is considerable, then a toric back surface or a bitoric lens should be considered in either a full aperture or lenticulated design.

9.8.1 Apex lenses

If a conventional corneal lens decentres, or the pupil is markedly eccentric, or the corneal toricity is excessive, then the apex lens of Fraser and Gordon [7] may be worth consideration. Its design is very similar to that of the fenestrated lens for optic measurement (FLOM) but it is thinner and smaller without the abrupt transition which is replaced by an intermediate curve.

In order to keep the lens as thin as possible, a lenticulated design is essential. A total diameter between 12 and 14 mm with a BOZD of around 9 mm seems to be typical, although the dimensions for an individual eye appear to be decided by intuition based on experience. If the lens is made from PMMA, it will need a number of fenestrations to meet the corneal demand for oxygen. The oxygen transmission may be further improved by using a gas permeable material.

9.8.2 Rigid gas permeable lenses (RGPs)

A gas-permeable lens for an aphake will have a large centre thickness and this will limit the degree of oxygen transmission. The contact lens practitioner will therefore, need to work as precisely as possible. It is unreasonable to expect the permeability of the material to compensate for any shortcomings in the fitting relationship between the contact lens and the cornea. Indeed, this is a philosophy that should be extended to the fitting of RGP lenses to any eye. The idea that the cornea will tolerate an unusually large and/or steep lens because the lens is made from a gas-permeable material should be discouraged.

The improved compatibility of the cornea and the RGP lens may arise from factors other than the permeability of the material. It is worth remembering the remarkable improvement that occurred in patients suffering corneal oedema with PMMA lenses when these patients were transferred to cellulose acetate butyrate (CAB) lenses, which had very limited permeability.

9.9 Soft lenses

The soft lens is, in many ways, an attractive proposition for the aphakic patient. There is less chance of mechanical insult of the relatively insensitive cornea. Also, centration problems are likely to be less than those of a corneal hard or RGP lens. The large BOZD of the soft lens will minimize problems of flare.

The lens for an aphake will be around 0.5 mm larger than that required for the routine patient. A lenticular design will be essential to keep the lens thickness within acceptable limits.

The lens material should be one which is resistant to dehydration because the ageing eye is often deficient in its lachrymal supply. In routine contact lens fitting, it is suggested that the practitioner avoids using very thin, or high water content, lenses where there is a dry-eye condition. This recommendation is at odds with the need to provide adequate corneal oxygenation. When dehydration occurs, the lens fit will tighten and the lens will be more susceptible to surface deposit formation. It has to be said that contact lenses, particularly soft contact lenses, and dry eyes are not a good combination.

Lens handling problems, which are likely with both old and very young patients, make the extended-wear regime worthy of consideration.

9.10 Extended wear

Extended wear is a particularly attractive proposition when a patient is elderly, hyperopic and totally presbyopic. This combination of features leads inevitably to lens handling difficulties which may be insurmountable. It must also be noted that the long-term effects of extended wear, which are largely unknown, are of little significance to the elderly patient.

9.10.1 Extended-wear soft lenses

The practitioner should note that the track record of extended-wear soft lenses strongly suggests that this is the most risky mode of contact lens wear. There is an increased possibility of complications arising which may produce permanent corneal damage. Graham *et al.* [8] demonstrated that aphakes are at a higher risk of incurring sight-threatening infections than other extended-wear groups. They found a 55% incidence of serious complications in extended-wear aphakic patients, compared with an 8.8% incidence for daily-wear aphakes. They concluded that daily lens wear is a viable alternative to the IOL for aphakes under the age of 70. For older patients, dexterity problems and the risks associated with extended wear suggest that a spectacle correction should be given serious consideration, before opting for extended-wear contact lenses. The Oxford cataract team [9] compared aphakic patients wearing PMMA lenses on a daily basis with those wearing soft lenses on an extended-wear basis and noted that the extended-wear group required more lens replacements, more follow-up visits and had more serious complications. Also, cessation of lens wear was more common in the extended-wear group. They concluded that contact lens wear still provides a viable alternative to the IOL. Ulcerative keratitis was found to be seven times more likely in the extended-wear aphakes examined by Glynn *et al.* [10] than their daily-wear counterparts. It was also noted that daily-wear aphakes were six times more likely to develop ulcerative keratitis than daily-wear cosmetic lens wearers. The prevalence of corneal vascularization in aphakic patients using soft lenses on an extended-wear basis is around 14% which is considerably higher than that for cosmetic lens wearers. Surface deposits may develop more rapidly because of the thicker lens substance and the probability of age-related tear dysfunction.

For some patients, extended wear may be the only feasible option. An example would be the very young congenital aphake, where the risks of contact lens wear must be offset against the positive advantage of minimizing amblyopic complications. There is, however, nothing to stop a competent relative or friend accepting the responsibility for inserting, removing and disinfecting the contact lenses of an aphakic patient of any age. It is obvious from the above that, as always, we must consider each case on its individual merits. It can be pointed out, for example, that male aphakic patients have a better success rate than female patients, probably because of the motivation arising from maintaining employment and/or his driving licence. Also, it may be advisable to prescribe two pairs of lenses for all aphakes because the loss ratio for the aphakic patient is about one third higher than for patients with more routine refractive errors.

Generally, the use of extended-wear soft lenses is a costly exercise. The lenses may suffer from rapid surface deposition, which means that frequent replacement is necessary. The frequent aftercare checks required are time consuming, and serious complications arising during wear are a distinct possibility.

9.10.2 Silicone elastomer lenses

The use of high-permeability materials is desirable because lens thickness works against good oxygen transmission. Silicone elastomer lenses may therefore be considered appropriate both on this account and also because they will not dehydrate in a dry eye. Baker [11] concluded

that silicone elastomer lenses are easier to insert and are more likely to remain in the eye, thereby reducing the rate of lens loss. The tolerance to these lenses appears to be better in children than in adults. In general, the corneas stay clear but surface deposits on the lenses may be a problem.

9.10.3 Rigid gas-permeable extended-wear lenses

The use of RGP corneal lenses on an extended-wear basis for aphakic eyes is finding favour with some practitioners. Garcia *et al.* [12] claim a 67% success rate using extended-wear RGPs (CAB, Boston or Paraperm) with 186 patients. It must be noted that two of these patients developed corneal ulcers. High-permeability materials are theoretically more attractive because of the substantial lens thickness. As with daily wear, a larger than normal lens total diameter may be required to ensure adequate centring and pupil coverage. A lenticulated design will ensure that the lens thickness is minimized. When compared with the soft lens, the RGP is:

(a) more robust;
(b) less troubled by surface deposits and easier to clean;
(c) able to correct corneal astigmatism more effectively;
(d) more likely to be physiologically compatible with the cornea because of the higher permeability, smaller lens thickness and smaller total diameter.

9.11 Scleral lenses

The one remaining lens type worth mentioning is the scleral lens. Scleral lenses are very robust and provide a physical protective barrier for the eye during wear. The tear layer trapped between the lens and cornea prevents drying of the anterior eye, even in dry-eyed patients. Their sheer size makes them easier to handle in some respects and certainly makes them more difficult to lose. Correction of high degrees of astigmatism presents few problems and the incorporation of a prism at any base–apex orientation is possible. The optic zone can be specifically sited if necessary over a postoperatively decentred pupil. Elderly aphakes generally appear to tolerate scleral lenses very well. Some will be content with short wearing periods because most of their day is spent in a sedentary manner, where a spectacle correction will be acceptable. As already mentioned elsewhere, it is likely that the cornea of an aphakic eye exhibits less hypoxic change when subjected to contact lens wear and so a prolonged wearing time may be easier to achieve. The advantages of making a scleral lens in RGP material are obvious and the investigations involving RGP scleral lenses are encouraging. However, their substantial centre thickness increases the shape factor of the lens and thereby increases the retinal image size (see Section 8.8.2). This means that the scleral lens is less suited to correction of the monocular aphakic patient.

9.12 Contact lens correction of the young aphake

Young aphakic patients will have suffered either congenital or traumatic cataract which will be either unilateral or bilateral.

The corneal diameter will have reached almost adult proportions in a 1-year-old infant, but the corneal radius is likely to be steeper than the typical adult value. The corneal physiology is similar to that of the adult and the topography is only slightly altered by the surgery because lensectomy and aspiration are the most common procedures and the small scars which remain induce minimal astigmatism.

Infants born with bilateral congenital cataracts should be operated on and optically corrected as soon as possible, to minimize amblyopic complications. It is most likely that soft extended-wear lenses will be fitted for comfort and convenience after consultation with an ophthalmologist. Amaya *et al.* [13] achieved an 85% success rate over a 3-year period and concluded that soft lens correction was safe, versatile and cost effective. Epstein *et al.* [14] found no significant difference in endothelial cell density or polymegathism, when they compared ten aphakic children wearing extended-wear soft lenses with nine unoperated control children. It must be said, however, that this is an unusual result, considering the extensively documented adverse effects of daily-wear soft lenses on the endothelium. Edmonds [15] advocates the use of a suitable soft lens with an aggressive extended wear schedule, in order to

combat the amblyopia problem in very young children. Once the child is old enough to handle the lenses effectively, then a daily-wear regime is more desirable. It is thus advisable to convert to a daily-wear regime as soon as this is a practical proposition. It is appropiate from the outset to encourage the parents to get used to inserting, removing and disinfecting the lenses.

The options available to the practitioner are soft lenses (particularly high water content lenses), silicone rubber lenses, high-permeability RGP lenses and scleral lenses.

The refraction must rely totally on retinoscopy but cycloplegic eye drops should not be necessary. If the correcting lens is hand held before the eye, the vertex distance will be variable and difficult to measure with any precision. It is advisable to keep the vertex distance as small as possible in order to give a spectacle correction that is more nearly equal to the contact lens refraction. Where a trial lens can be fitted, an over refraction should be performed with a high plus contact lens *in situ*, and the vertex distance will then have little influence on the result. The BVP required for the contact lens will be in the region of +30.00 D to correct the eye for distance. Babies are interested in objects generally within arms length and so an overcorrection of the order of +2.00 to +3.00 D may be appropriate. The high plus contact lens is inevitably thick, and consequently corneal hypoxia is likely, even with oxygen-permeable materials. This can be minimized by using a lenticular design with the smallest acceptable FOZD. The carrier zone and the junction will, however, have to be thicker than in an adult lens to maintain some robustness. It is not advisable to attempt to correct any residual astigmatism by using toric lenses. The practitioner should determine the best sphere as accurately as possible using a non-toric lens design. It is usually not possible to take the keratometry readings and so it may be best to assume that the corneal curvature will be around 7.2 mm.

9.12.1 Soft lenses

In the case of the soft lens, a high water content material should be used on young infants because they spend much of the day asleep. If the material does not stand up to the wear and tear, then a lower water content material, which should be more robust, can be considered when the child is older. It is worth noting that the manufacturers of some of the high water content lenses claim a high level of durability.

The corneal diameter of the infant is a little smaller than that of the adult, so a soft lens total diameter is typically around 12.50 mm. In some cases, a larger lens is required because of decentration problems.

It is desirable to provide lenses from stock at the end of the first visit and this means having each specification duplicated in the fitting set. It is also advisable to provide the patient with a spare pair of lenses which further doubles the size of the fitting set. The large fitting set required means that it is appropriate that the infant is fitted by a practitioner who specializes in this type of patient, and consequently this is more likely to be an exercise performed in a hospital eye department.

Obviously conventional fitting assessment techniques cannot be used and the practitioner must improvise in her or his assessment of lens fit.

9.12.2 Silicone elastomer lenses

Where soft lenses are unsuccessful for any reason, the practitioner should consider the possibility of transferring to silicone rubber lenses. These lenses may be difficult to remove and their surfaces degrade rapidly. For both soft and silicone rubber lenses it is better to err towards a loose rather than a tight fit.

9.12.3 Rigid gas-permeable lenses

RGP lenses need to be fitted under general anaesthesia in order to acquire keratometry readings and to assess the fluorescein picture. Slightly older children may be co-operative enough to allow this without recourse to an anaesthetic. The lens total diameter is typically around 9 mm, so that the lens appears to be rather large on the cornea when compared with the fit of an adult eye.

9.12.4 Scleral lenses

The scleral lens can only be fitted under general anaesthesia, usually using the impression technique. The distinct possibility of a limited wearing time for PMMA material must be considered along with the advantages of dura-

bility, size, physical protection, absence of deposits, stability of vision and simple disinfection. Its ability to provide clearance of any corneal scars which would complicate the fitting of other lens types must also be considered. The limited wearing time problem can be minimized by fenestrations, channels and/or manufacturing the lens from a gas-permeable material.

9.12.5 Optical correction

For all lens types, as the child gets older, the power requires adjustment in order to compensate for increasing object distances. Ultimately the contact lens will be powered for distance correction but there must also obviously be a facility for near correction. This could take the form of reading spectacles, bifocal contact lenses or a monovision system, where one eye is corrected for distance and the fellow eye for near. The latter option must be considered with caution, since it may encourage the breakdown of binocular vision in a young child. It may also be necessary to correct the astigmatism fully once the child starts to attend school. This could be achieved using a supplementary pair of bifocal spectacles if the practitioner is reluctant to interfere with an otherwise successful contact lens correction. The provision of a spare pair of contact lenses has already been mentioned but the provision of a back-up pair of spectacles which can be used if the contact lenses are not worn for any reason is also recommended.

Unilateral aphakes must be encouraged to use the aphakic eye by occluding the fellow eye for a considerable part of each day if amblyopia is to be avoided. In the case of traumatic aphakes, it is necessary to monitor the cornea with extra care because neovascularization is more likely in the presence of scar tissue.

9.13 Aftercare

The two most obvious differences between the aphakic and the average contact lens wearer are the reduction in corneal sensitivity produced by the surgery and the degree of difficulty encountered in handling the contact lenses. On the positive side, however, there are fewer worries about the long-term consequences of contact lens wear in the elderly patient. Elderly patients may require timely reminders for their aftercare appointments, and the need for adequate ophthalmological follow-up must be emphasized to them. It is appropriate to request that the patient demonstrates their lens handling abilities and that the patient also demonstrates the techniques that they use for cleaning and disinfection, in order that the practitioner can be assured that the procedures are adequate.

The likelihood of a dry-eye condition would be expected to be accompanied by a lens deposit problem, and this appears to be the case with the aphake. Thus, inspection of the lenses both on and off the eye is particularly important. In general, the deposits will be most obvious when the lenses are out of the eyes, using dark field illumination. The only change that will be most obvious with a light background is lens discoloration.

A major problem encountered with all soft lens wearers, which unfortunately arises all too frequently, is that of corneal vascularization. In the aphakic patient, neovascularization is more, rather than less, likely and causes the practitioner a dilemma when it is observed. It can be argued that any neovascularization is unacceptable but this attitude would condemn the patient to a spectacle correction. If, on the other hand, it is decided to accept a certain amount of neovascularization, then a question mark hangs over the degree allowable and this appears to be a matter of opinion. It is then a case of weighing the benefits against the risks. It could perhaps, be dealt with by more effective monitoring, achieved by more frequent after care visits. Alternatively, ophthalmological advice could be sought in order to resolve this aspect of patient management.

Recommended reading

Douthwaite, W. A. *Contact Lens Optics*, Butterworths, London (1987)

Phillips, A. J. and Stone, J. *Contact Lenses*, 3rd edn, Butterworths, London (1989)

References

1. Port, M.J.A. The spectral transmission of contact lenses. *Contax*, September, 13–16 (1986)
2. Mandell, R.B. *Contact Lens Practice*, Charles Thomas, Springfield, pp. 353–364 (1968)
3. Guillon, M. and Warland, J. Aniseikonia and binocular function in unilateral aphakes wearing contact lenses. *Journal of the British Contact Lens Association*, **3**, 36–38 (1980)
4. Osamu, K., Yoshitaka, M., Tatsuo, H., Hiroko, O. and Isamu, A. Binocular function in unilateral aphakia. *Ophthalmology*, **95**, 1088–1093 (1988)
5. Douthwaite, W.A., Ford, M.W., Francis, J.L. and Stone, J. Practical optics and computer design of contact lenses. In *Contact Lenses*, 3rd edn (edited by J.L. Phillips and J. Stone), Butterworths, London, p. 208 (1980)
6. Bennett, A.G. Power changes of soft contact lenses due to bending. *Ophthalmic Optician*, **16**, 939–945 (1976)
7. Fraser, J.P. and Gordon, S.P. The apex lens for uniocular aphakia. *Ophthalmic Optician*, **7**, 1190–1194, 1247-1253 (1967)
8. Graham, C.M., Dart, J.K.G. and Buckley, R.J. Extended wear hydrogels and daily wear hard contact lenses for aphakia. Success and complications compared on a longitudinal study. *Ophthalmology*, **3**, 1489–1494 (1986)
9. Oxford Cataract Treatment and Evaluation Team. The use of contact lenses to correct aphakia in a clinical trial of cataract management. *Eye*, **4**, 138–144 (1990)
10. Glynn, R.J., Schein, O.D., Seddon, J.M., Poggio, E.C., Goodfellow, J.R., Scardino, V.A., Shannon, M.J. and Kenyon, K.R. The incidence of ulcerative keratitis among aphakic contact lens wearers in New England. *Archives of Ophthalmology*, **109**, 104–107 (1991)
11. Baker, J.D. Visual rehabilitation of aphakic children: contact lenses. *Ophthalmology*, **34**, 366–371 (1990).
12. Garcia, G.E., Aucoin, J. and Gladstone, G. Extended wear rigid gas permeable lenses used for correction of aphakia. *CLAO Journal*, **16**, 195–199 (1990)
13. Amaya, L., Speedwell, L. and Taylor, D. Contact lenses for infant aphakia. *British Journal of Ophthalmology*, **74**, 150–154 (1990)
14. Epstein, R.J., Fernandes, A. and Gammon, J.A. The correction of aphakia in infants with hydrogel extended wear contact lenses. *Ophthalmology*, **95**, 1102–1106 (1988)
15. Edmonds, S.A. Contact lens management of aphakic children. *Contact Lens Forum*, **15**, 15–18 (1990)

The intraocular lens

William A. Douthwaite

10.1 Correction by intraocular lens (IOL)

As an alternative to a spectacle or contact lens correction, an IOL can be considered as an increasingly common alternative form of correction. An eye which is fitted with an IOL is said to be pseudophakic. It is worth noting here that, as with any other form of correction, the IOL should contain an ultraviolet (UV) absorber in order to protect the retina from harmful radiation. The crystalline lens normally absorbs the UV radiation around 315–390 nm. The typical IOL containing a UV absorber will exhibit a 10% transmission cut off at 400 nm.

There have been three main types of implant.

(a) Anterior chamber, where the implant is fixed in front of the iris, by the haptic resting in the anterior angle. This type is easy to position and rarely dislocates. It can be used after intracapsular or extracapsular extraction. It is used when an aphakic eye previously corrected by spectacles or contact lenses is to have an IOL fitted.
(b) Iris supported, where the IOL is attached by loops to the anterior and posterior iris surface. Figure 10.1 shows a typical iris-supported IOL. The loops may irritate the iris leading to inflammation and iris atrophy.
(c) Posterior chamber. This lies behind the iris and is fixed by struts extending into the capsule after extracapsular extraction of the crystalline lens. Within about 2 months of the operation, the lens becomes fixed by fibrosis and the pupil may be dilated when required. This type of IOL is in the best optical position because it most nearly corresponds to the position of the crystalline lens which it has replaced. Also the posterior-chamber position removes the risk of damage to the corneal endothelium which is a possibility with the other two types. Figure 10.2 shows two typical posterior-chamber IOLs.

Most IOLs are of the posterior-chamber type and are fitted with the posterior lens capsule intact, after extracapsular extraction of the cataract. IOLs usually possess a 5–6 mm optic zone which is centred by the supports (haptic zone). A significant number of patients develop opacification of the lens capsule within 3–5 years, resulting in reduced visual acuity (VA). Capsulotomy with a YAG laser restores vision, but it is not entirely without risk. Transient increase in the intraocular pressure can occur, and poor focusing of the laser might produce some pitting or crazing of the IOL which does not usually affect the vision.

Implantation of an IOL was introduced in the 1950s. The early problems have been addressed and it is now a routine and often preferred approach in the surgical treatment of cataract. The use of a standard IOL of fixed power resulted in a large variation in postoperative refractive error with unexpected results in some

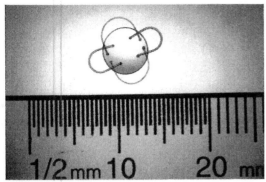

Figure 10.1 An iris-supported IOL.

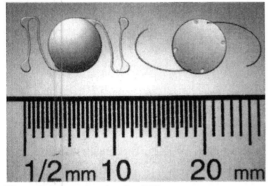

Figure 10.2 Posterior-chamber IOLs.

The crystalline lens power shows no correlation with the refractive error of the eye. Emmctropic eyes possess crystalline lenses with powers varying from +15.00 to +24.00 D. The mean power is around +19.70 D [1].

The anterior chamber IOL is in a more anterior position than the crystalline lens and so its power requires some modification to compensate for the change in position. A power around +18.00 D would be appropriate. The majority of patients are elderly, spending most of their time indoors, and so it may be appropriate to leave them around 1.00 to 2.00 D myopic. This will help them with middle distance and close work. So a recommendation for a standard lens power is around +19.50 D.

A number of workers have compared postoperative refractive results between patients with standard-power IOLs and those with IOLs of a power calculated to correct each individual refractive error. The consensus appears to show that the calculated group produced better uncorrected vision.

10.2 Estimation of IOL power from refractive error

If we consider that a +18.00 D lens will correct a previously emmetropic eye, then we will need to add more positive power to the IOL for hyperopes and less positive power for myopes. The refractive error of the eye may change as a result of the developing cataract (usually in a more myopic direction) and so the principle described above applies to the refractive error before cataract development. Binkhorst [2] suggested that the IOL power should be changed by 1.25 D for every 1.00 D of refractive error. Other workers have suggested that the change in refractive error and the change in IOL power should be equal. Alternatively another group concluded that the patient would be most content with 2.00 D of myopia applied to the latter approach. Thus, to summarize, if we consider an eye which was 3.00 D hyperopic before the cataract developed, we could give it:

(a) the standard +19.50 D lens;
(b) the IOL power deduced using Binkhorst's recommendation, which gives +18.00 + 3.75 = +21.75 D;
(c) the alternative of equal changes in IOL power and refractive error giving +18.00 + 3.00 = +21.00 D;
(d) the application of the same rule as (c) with a 2.00 D myopic shift giving +18.00 + 3.00 + 2.00 = +23.00 D.

It might, therefore, be appropriate to go for a power at the centre of the range defined above which is +21.25 D, and this suggests that option (c) may be the best. However, this simplistic approach has been shown to produce results little better than using a standard-power IOL. In order to improve upon the precision of the determination of the IOL power, it is necessary to measure and record:

(a) the power of the cornea;
(b) the depth of the anterior chamber (ACD);
(c) the axial length of the eye.

See Figure 10.3.

10.3 Calculation of the IOL power

If we know the axial length of the eye, the ACD and the radius of curvature of the cornea, then

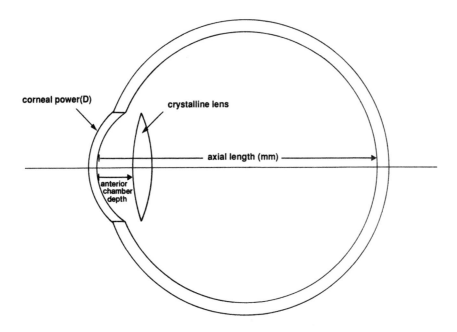

Figure 10.3 The measurements required for the calculation of the power of the IOL.

we can, by using the step-along method, calculate the theoretical power of the IOL. Figure 10.4 illustrates the path of light rays through a typical pseudophakic eye. The negative spectacle lens is there to remind the reader that the surgeon may be aiming for low myopia (as an alternative to emmetropia) in order to help with middle distance and close work. The assumption made in this example is that the negative spectacle lens is producing an incident vergence, at the anterior cornea (vergence ①) of -1.50 D. From a practical point of view, this would be achieved by a -1.50 D spectacle lens because the 12 mm vertex distance would have no significant effect on the effective power of the lens at the eye. In fact the effective power of a -1.50 D lens at the eye is 0.027 D less negative for a 12 mm vertex distance.

10.3.1 The cornea

Let us suppose the keratometer has given a radius of curvature of 7.80 mm for the anterior cornea in our example. If we take the constants of Gullstrand's number one schematic eye, then we can make the assumption that the corneal thickness is 0.5 mm and the posterior surface radius is 88% of the anterior surface radius. This

gives a posterior surface radius of 6.86 mm (to two decimal places).

Thus the power of the anterior cornea is

$$\frac{n_c - 1}{r_1} = \frac{376}{7.8}$$
$$= +48.21 \text{ D}$$

and the power of the posterior cornea is

$$\frac{n_a - n_c}{r_2} = \frac{-40}{6.86}$$
$$= -5.83 \text{ D}$$

We can now use the step-along method illustrated in Figure 10.5.

	Vergence (D)	Distance (mm)
① =	-1.50	
F_1 =	-48.21 (add)	

$$② = +46.71 \rightarrow \frac{1000}{46.71} \rightarrow 21.41$$

$$00.36 \quad t/n_c \text{ (subtract)}$$

$$③ = +47.51 \leftarrow \frac{1000}{21.05} \leftarrow 21.05$$

$$F_2 = -5.83 \text{ (add)}$$

$$④ = +41.68$$

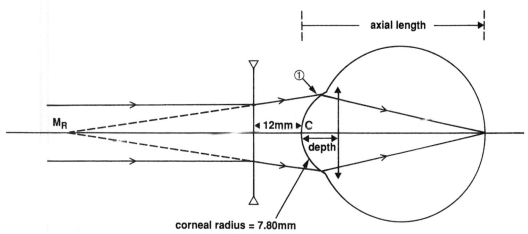

Figure 10.4 Path of the light rays through the pseudophakic eye. ① represents the incident vergence on the cornea, which is the reciprocal of the distance $M_R C$ in metres.

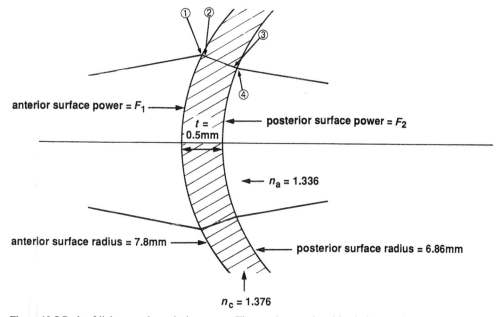

Figure 10.5 Path of light rays through the cornea. The numbers enclosed in circles are the vergence labels.

10.3.2 The emergent vergence from the IOL

Let us assume that the measurement of the ACD is 3.5 mm, combined with the corneal thickness of 0.5 mm, and we intend to use a plano-convex IOL of centre thickness 0.7 mm and refractive index 1.417. The axial length measurement is 24 mm, so that we can now deduce the distance from the posterior lens surface to the retina. This is

$$24 - (0.5 + 3.5 + 0.7) = 19.3 \text{ mm}$$

(see Figure 10.6). Thus vergence ⑧ must be $(1.336/19.3) \times 1000$ if the light rays are to focus on the retina, which is $+69.22$ D.

10.3.3 Cornea to posterior surface of IOL

We must now continue with the step-along method from vergence ④ until we calculate vergence ⑦. The algebraic subtraction of vergence ⑧ from vergence ⑦ will give the surface power of the posterior surface of the IOL *in situ*.

Vergence (D)	Distance (mm)

$$④ = +41.68 \rightarrow \frac{1000}{41.68} \rightarrow 23.99$$

$$02.62 \quad t/n_a$$

(subtract)

$$⑤ = +46.79 \leftarrow \frac{1000}{21.37} \leftarrow 21.37$$

$$F_3 = +00.00 \quad \text{(add)}$$

$$⑥ = +46.79 \rightarrow \frac{1000}{46.79} \rightarrow 21.37$$

$$00.49 \quad t/n_1 \text{ (subtract)}$$

$$⑦ = +47.89 \leftarrow \frac{1000}{20.88} \leftarrow 20.88$$

Surface power $F_4 = ⑧ - ⑦ = +69.22 - 47.89$

$$= +21.33 \text{ D}$$

The back surface power of a plano-convex lens (back surface convex) will also be the back vertex power (BVP) and the equivalent power of the lens. Therefore the IOL BVP is $+21.33$ D in the eye and this is also the equivalent power.

The radius of curvature of this back surface can be calculated using:

$$r = \frac{n_v - n_1}{F}$$

$$= \frac{-81}{21.33}$$

$$= -3.80 \text{ mm}$$

The power of this surface in air

$$= \frac{1 - n_1}{r}$$

$$= \frac{-417}{-3.8}$$

$$= +109.74 \text{ D}$$

This is also the BVP and the equivalent power of the IOL in air.

The above exercise is a tedious one, particularly if repeated calculations are required. It does, however, lend itself very readily to computerization because computers will happily perform these tedious calculations over and over again and they will do it very quickly.

10.4 Retinal image size with an implant

10.4.1 Image size corrected

Referring to Figure 8.5 (in Section 8.7) and assuming our eye views a distant object which subtends an angle θ, the final image size h_3', for a system which has one thin spectacle lens and an eye with four refracting surfaces, as in Figure 10.6, will be:

$$h_3' = f_1 \tan \theta \times \frac{①}{②} \times \frac{③}{④} \times \frac{⑤}{⑥} \times \frac{⑦}{⑧}$$

where f_1 is the focal length of the spectacle lens and θ is the angle subtended at the eye by the object.

Thus $f_1 = \frac{1000}{-1.5} = -666.67$ mm

$$h_3' = -666.67 \tan \theta \times \frac{-1.5}{46.71} \times \frac{47.51}{41.68} \times \frac{46.79}{46.79} \times \frac{47.8}{69.2}$$

$$= -666.67 \tan \theta \times 0.0253251 = -16.88 \tan \theta$$

10.4.2 Image size in emmetropia

Suppose the initially emmetropic eye views the same distant object (see Figure 10.7):

Vergence (D)	Distance (mm)

$$② = +48.21 \rightarrow \frac{1000}{48.21} \rightarrow 20.74$$

$$00.36 \quad t/n_c$$
(subtract)

$$③ = +49.07 \leftarrow \frac{1000}{20.38} \leftarrow 20.38$$

$$F_2 = -05.83 \text{ (add)}$$

$$④ = +43.24 \rightarrow \frac{1000}{43.24} \rightarrow 23.13$$

$$02.62 \quad t/n_a$$
(subtract)

$$⑤ = +48.76 \leftarrow \frac{1000}{20.51} \leftarrow 20.51$$

$$F_3 = +08.50 \text{ (add)}$$

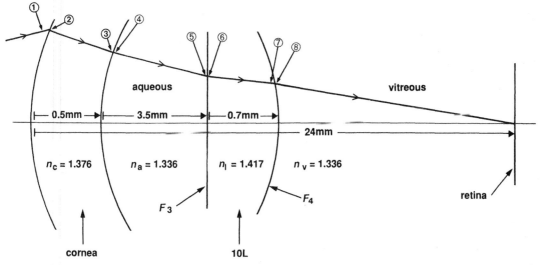

Figure 10.6 Passage of light through the pseudophakic eye. The numbers in circles are vergence labels.

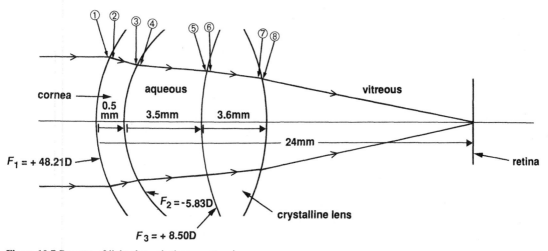

Figure 10.7 Passage of light through the emmetropic eye.

⑥ $= +57.26 \rightarrow \dfrac{1000}{57.26} \rightarrow 17.46$

$\qquad\qquad\qquad\qquad 02.54 \quad t/n_1$

$\qquad\qquad\qquad\qquad \overline{\qquad\qquad}$ (subtract)

⑦ $= +67.02 \leftarrow \dfrac{1000}{14.92} \leftarrow 14.92$

The distance between the posterior lens surface and the retina is: $24 - (0.5 + 3.5 + 3.6) = 16.4$ mm (see Figure 10.7).

Therefore vergence ⑧ must be

$$\dfrac{1.336}{16.4} \times 1000 = +81.46 \text{ D}$$

Retinal image size in emmetropia

$$h_e' = f_1 \tan \theta \times \dfrac{③}{④} \times \dfrac{⑤}{⑥} \times \dfrac{⑦}{⑧}$$

where f_1 is the focal length of the anterior corneal surface which is

$$-\dfrac{1000}{48.21} = -20.74 \text{ mm}$$

and θ is the angle subtended by the object at the eye.

Therefore

$$h_e' = -20.74 \tan \theta \times \frac{49.07}{43.24} \times \frac{48.76}{57.26} \times \frac{67.02}{81.46}$$

$$= -16.49 \tan \theta$$

A comparison of the retinal image sizes can now be made as follows:

$$\frac{h_3'}{h_e'} = \frac{-16.88}{-16.49}$$

$$= 1.024$$

Thus there is only a 2.4% increase in the retinal image size when the IOL is in place. Evidently, the IOL is the best optical correction in terms of the image size criterion, and binocular vision should be achieved with unilateral or bilateral pseudophakia.

10.5 Measurements required to calculate the power of the IOL

If the above calculations are going to be used in the clinical situation, it will be necessary to measure the axial length of the eye, the power of the cornea and the ACD.

10.5.1 Axial length measurement

This is the most important component in the calculation of IOL power [3,4]. It is currently measured by ultrasound techniques. Ultrasound consists of an acoustic wave made up of a series of compressions and rarefactions that can be propagated in fluids and solids. In the eye, it can be used to detect ocular and orbital abnormalities as well as to measure the ocular dimensions. The measurement of anatomical dimensions using ultrasound is called biometry. There are two basic types of ultrasound scanning used in the examination of the eye.

10.5.1.1 The A scan

This allows the examination of a thin slice through the tissues. It is the ultrasound equivalent of a slit-lamp optical section. The ultrasonic beam crosses a defined path within the eye and undergoes partial reflection at tissue boundaries. This is the method used for axial length measurement.

The A scan trace consists of a series of spikes that are viewed on an oscilloscope screen. Figure 10.8 illustrates a typical picture. The spikes occur where the beam passes from an area of one velocity to an area of different velocity. In the past, a small plastic water bath was fitted between the lids of an anaesthetized eye and was filled with gonioscopy fluid. The probe was positioned in the fluid without coming into direct contact with the cornea. Direct applanation of the probe on to the cornea was not recommended as the resulting indentation was believed to produce a prediction for axial length which was shorter than that produced when no direct contact occurred [3]. The present thinking on this issue is that the water bath is redundant and the probe is applied directly to the cornea. The ultrasonic beam must be aligned exactly with the visual axis to give a good result. When this occurs the spikes display maximum amplification and are all of nearly the same height [3,5,6].

Longstaff [7] showed that when the beam is 5° off axis, the error in alignment induces a 0.3 mm change in axial length. Therefore ultrasound units should, ideally, incorporate fixation targets in the probe to assist in accurate alignment, although most commercial instruments do not possess this facility. The axial length is calculated by measuring the elapsed time between the spikes on the oscilloscope screen. This is halved because the trace is produced by the wave returning to the probe. It is then necessary to multiply the time measurement by the speed of the beam in the tissues (1532 ms^{-1} for the aqueous and the vitreous; 1641 ms^{-1} for the lens). Hoffer [3] compared the results of using the above speeds with the results produced by assuming an average speed of 1550 ms^{-1}. The two approaches were in good agreement, and the single-speed approach was recommended. It is worth noting that the speed of the beam in the cataractous lens is very variable. It has been suggested that a small correction factor of 0.26 mm should be added to the axial length to account for the distance from the vitreoretinal surface to Bruch's membrane. Hoffer [8] compared IOL power calculations with and without this correction and found that incorporating the correction factor produced a result that was worse rather than better. It is therefore usually ignored.

An error of 0.1 mm in axial length measurement results in an optical error for the refractive

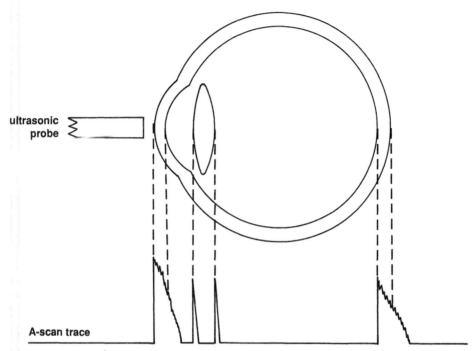

Figure 10.8 A schematic drawing of the principle of the A scan.

correction of around 0.25 D in the pseudophakic eye [1,3,9]. Thus, a number of axial length measurements should be taken, and, ideally, these should be found to vary by less than 0.1 mm.

10.5.1.2 The B scan

The electronic transducer is scanned across the eye and an image of the scanned ocular and orbital tissues can be constructed from the echoes. This technique is not used to determine axial length (see Section 6.8 for more details).

10.5.2 Measurement of corneal power

An aphakic eye can be regarded as a simple optical system where the total refracting power is produced by the cornea alone. If the power of the cornea and the axial length of the eye are known, then the calculation of the IOL power can be accomplished [6].

The keratometer is the instrument that is used clinically to measure the radius of curvature of the cornea. It does this by measuring the size of an image formed by reflection from an annular area of cornea of approximate diameter 3 mm, centred on the keratometric pole.

The power scale of the keratometer converts radius into power using:

$$F = \frac{n-1}{r}$$

where n (refractive index) is usually given a value of 1.3375 in order to predict the refractive power of the whole cornea (anterior and posterior corneal surfaces combined). It must be noted, however, that some keratometers use alternative values for the assumed refractive index. If a keratometer power scale has been derived using the 1.3375 value for refractive index, a radius reading of 7.5 mm will give a power of 45.00 D.

Where an eye undergoes the triple procedure of penetrating keratoplasty, cataract extraction and IOL implantation, the calculation of the IOL power is more difficult, as the mean keratometer reading of the postoperative cornea is not known before the operation. It is often impossible to obtain the original keratometer reading before the operation. Katz and Forster [10] suggest that keratometry should be attempted, and, where this fails, the keratometer should be used on the fellow eye.

The accuracy of keratometry in a normal implantation operation depends on the observer and the instrument. Binkhorst [6] suggests that the radius could be in error by as much as 0.2 mm or 1.00 D. Of more concern is the possibility that the radius may be changed by the surgical technique. Binkhorst [1] suggested altering the value of the refractive index of the cornea to compensate for the postoperative increase in the radius of curvature which he claims is 0.08 mm (0.50 D). Hoffer [3] estimated a flattening of 0.16 D in aphakic and 0.03 D in pseudophakic eyes, which is such a small change that it can be discounted in the IOL power calculation. However, probably the best advice that can be offered is for all surgeons to calculate their mean surgical change in corneal curvature and to incorporate the change into subsequent calculations.

Thus the keratometer suffers from some limitations. The widely accepted error in keratometer radius readings is 0.1 mm, which will produce a power error around 0.50 D in the spectacle correction of the pseudophakic eye. It must be emphasized that the keratometer measures the radius of curvature of a restricted annular region of the anterior corneal surface and, applying a number of assumptions, the power of the central cornea (anterior and posterior surfaces combined) is estimated. These assumptions may, or may not, be valid.

10.5.3 Measurement of the power of the IOL

The keratometer can be used to measure the power of an IOL by using it to measure the radius of curvature of the IOL surfaces and then converting the readings to surface power, using the refractive index of the IOL material. This is usually 1.417.

So the surface power in air is

$$\frac{n-1}{r} = \frac{417}{k \text{ reading (mm)}}$$

and the surface power in aqueous is

$$\frac{1417 - 1336}{k \text{ reading (mm)}}$$

The above applies to the anterior surface power.

In the case of the posterior surface, the numerator of the fraction adopts a negative sign (assuming a refractive index of 1.336 for the vitreous), and this, combined with the negative radius of the posterior surface of a lens, like that

in Figure 10.6, results in a positive power. If the lens is assumed to be thin, the surface powers are simply added together algebraically. If the lens is considered to be thick, the step-along method can be used to deduce both front and back vertex powers. It can be noted that the majority of IOLs are plano-convex in form, and, where the posterior surface is the curved surface, then, as already mentioned, the power of this surface is also the BVP of the lens.

10.5.4 Measurement of ACD

An assessment of the ACD is required to predict the position of the IOL in the eye in order to enable the exact implant power to be calculated. The ACD is the least important of the ocular dimensions required to calculate the power of the IOL. The pseudophakic ACD depends mainly on the anatomy of the iris root, the basic cataract-removal procedure, the design of the IOL and its method of attachment [11]. It is therefore likely that the ACD will be different in the pre- and post-operative states. Fyodorov *et al.* [12] describe a method of calculating the pseudophakic ACD by assuming that it will equal the sagitta of a circular arc. The radius of this arc is equal to the radius of curvature of the cornea, over a chord which is 1 mm longer than the visible external diameter of the cornea, along the appropriate meridian. The sagitta is calculated using the standard sag equation:

$$\text{sag} = r - \sqrt{(r_2 - y_2)}$$

where r is the keratometer reading and y is the semidiameter of the cornea plus 0.5 mm. They found, by postoperative measurement, that the pseudophakic chamber depth was within 0.03 mm of the calculated values derived from the preoperative measurements in 146 eyes. Binkhorst [6] suggested applying average values for the pseudophakic ACD according to the type of IOL used. This gave a range of ACDs from 3.19 to 4.20 mm for the different designs of IOL in use at that time.

The position of the IOL within the eye was defined by Hoffer [3] as the measurement from the front surface of the cornea to the front surface of the lens implant. He suggested using an optical pachometer to measure the pre-operative ACD.

For a prepupillary IOL, where the measured ACD is less than 3 mm, a lens position of 3.1 ± 0.5 mm should be assumed. Where the

ACD is 3–3.5 mm, a lens position of 3.3 mm should be assumed or it should be assumed to be equal to the measured ACD. Where the ACD is greater than 3.5 mm, a lens position of 3.5 mm should be assumed. For anterior and posterior chamber IOLs, lens positions of 3.3 and 4.0 mm respectively should be assumed.

When estimating the postoperative ACD, an error of 0.1 mm produces an error around 0.10 D in the spectacle correction of a pseudophakic eye, according to Binkhorst [6]. Hoffer [3] enlarged on this by suggesting that a 1 mm error in the position of the IOL produces a 0.25 D error in implant power in an eye with a long axial length and an error of 1.00 D in an eye with an axial length in the normal range. If the eye has a short axial length, the error increases further to around 2.50 D.

10.6 Theoretical formulae

Formulae that use geometrical optical principles to calculate the IOL power required in an individual eye were first published by Fyodorov and Kolinko in 1967 [13]. Colenbrander [14] derived a formula for the calculation of the power of an iris clip lens by considering the following:

(a) the refractive index of the aqueous and vitreous
(b) the power of the cornea
(c) the axial distance from the anterior corneal apex to the front surface of the IOL
(d) the axial length of the eye.

The relationship derived was as follows:

$$F_1 = \frac{n_1}{l - v - 0.00005} - \frac{n_1}{(n_1/F_c) - v - 0.00005}$$

where F_1 = power of iris clip lens; l = axial length; F_c = power of cornea; v = ACD; n_1 = refractive index of aqueous and vitreous. This basic approach was followed by others who devised alternative formulae. Thijessen [15], for example, used a schematic eye with optical properties based on those of Gullstrand and Le Grand. He simplified these by considering the cornea to be a single refracting surface and by assuming the crystalline lens to be thin. He devised a graph for reading off the IOL power required for emmetropia assuming an ACD of 3.5 mm (the generally accepted average value). Where the ACD is not 3.5 mm, the IOL power

should be adjusted by 1.50 D per mm difference. The graph consists of an x-axis of axial length and a y-axis of corneal radius of curvature which determine the power of the implant. He also emphasized that the axial length measurement should be as accurate as possible, if an exact calculation of the power of the IOL is to be of any practical value.

His formula is:

$$P_1 = \frac{n_v}{l - d_2 - (d_3 n_v/n_1)} - \frac{n_a}{(n_a/P_c) - d_2 + d_3}$$

where P_1 = power of the IOL; l = axial length; P_c = power of cornea; d_2 = ACD (IOL position); d_3 = IOL thickness; n_a = refractive index of aqueous; n_v = refractive index of vitreous; n_1 = refractive index of IOL.

Binkhorst [1] derived perhaps the most widely used formula to calculate the IOL power to render an eye emmetropic. This is:

$$D = \frac{1336(4r - a)}{(a - d)(4r - d)}$$

where D = power of the IOL (D) in fluid of refractive index 1.336 (aqueous and vitreous); r = radius of curvature of anterior cornea (mm); a = axial length (mm); d = axial distance from anterior corneal vertex to the anterior surface of the IOL (mm). This assumes a thin IOL and a refractive index of 4/3 for the cornea.

Fritz *et al.* [16] considered three of the popular formulae: (a) Binkhorst Loones; (b) Colenbrander; (c) Fyodorov, Linksz and Galin. They concluded that they are simply related after algebraic manipulation and they then have the same form:

$$P = \frac{n}{A - D - g_{(t)}} - \frac{n}{(n/K) - D - g_{(t)}}$$

where P = power of IOL; n = refractive index of aqueous; A = axial length; K = corneal power; D = ACD; $g_{(t)}$ = function of IOL thickness.

In fact, the difference in the calculated IOL power between any of the three equations is 0.10 D which is much less than the manufacturer's tolerances and the errors of axial length and curvature measurement.

10.7 The problem of the short eye

This is well documented. Clinical experience with ultrasound and the calculation formulae has revealed that the prediction of too strong an IOL power is common. The Binkhorst [1] formula calculates an IOL power that is always 0.50 D more powerful than other formulae. Hoffer [17], feels that some assumptions in Binkhorst's approach are not valid, i.e.:

(a) postoperative corneal flattening;
(b) post-operative shortening of axial length;
(c) retinal thickness compensation.

Shammas [18] addressed the problem of the short eye and suggested that a correction factor of -0.50 to -1.00 D should be added to the IOL power. He also noted that the calculated power results in a hyperopic error in large eyes, which should therefore incorporate a correction factor of around $+1.00$ D. He modified Colenbrander's formula by incorporating a correction factor which varies with axial length. The correction consists of 0.1 mm being added to the axial length for each 1 mm that the axial length is shorter than 23 mm, and subtracting 0.1 mm from the axial length for each 1 mm that the axial length is longer than 23 mm. Thus, the axial length becomes:

$$l - 0.1(l - 23)$$

where l is the measured axial length.

Shammas [18] claimed that these modifications yield a higher accuracy than the Binkhorst [1] or the Colenbrander [14] equations. However, he also noted that each formula yields the best results for the surgeon who derived it! The Shammas formula is:

$$P = \cfrac{1336}{l - 0.1(l - 23) - c - 0.005} - \cfrac{1}{(1.0125/K) - (c + 0.005)/1336}$$

where P = IOL power for emmetropia; l = axial length (mm); K = keratometer reading (mm); c = ACD (mm).

All the formulae have a similar structure with the differences between them being subtle. A number of errors arise using these optically determined formulae but they lend themselves readily to incorporation into simple computer programs or, perhaps more conveniently, into incorporation into a spreadsheet program. An alternative approach to the use of the above programs is to use regression formulae.

10.8 Regression formulae

Regression analysis is a method of deriving an equation to fit an assumed relationship between two variables. A linear regression relationship can be plotted using the method of least squares, which is a standard statistical technique incorporated into many pocket calculators. Loyd and Gills [19] developed the first linear regression equation in 1978. Retzlaff [20] derived the formula:

$$P = 116.6 - 2.4l - 0.8K$$

where P = IOL power for emmetropia; l = axial length (mm); K = keratometer reading (D). He claimed that this formula produces more accurate predictions than any of the methods described so far. This linear regression formula uses the uncorrected axial length measurement. The retinal thickness factor and the ACD are ignored. Regression formulae that include a correction factor for retinal thickness were found to produce poorer results.

Optical formulae must take into consideration the following values:

(a) postoperative ACD;
(b) corneal refractive index;
(c) aqueous and vitreous refractive index;
(d) the inclusion of the retinal thickness factor in relation to the axial length.

None of the above are included in a regression equation, although the equation will only apply to results found using a keratometer which has assumed the same corneal refractive index as the instrument used to determine the equation.

Sanders and Kraff [21] used multiple regression analysis which analyses the error in prediction accuracy, i.e. the residual refractive error on completion and the best linear equation is found to determine the implant power for postoperative emmetropia. The axial length was found to be the most important parameter in terms of its influence on the result, followed by keratometry, with measurement of the ACD affecting the prediction accuracy of the formula by less than 1%. The best-fit formula found is of the form:

IOL power = $(A + B \times$ axial length$) + (C \times$ keratometry power)

where $A = 124$, $B = -2.74$ and $C = -0.97$ for the Shearing-style anterior-chamber lens (IOLAB).

This formula can be used for other implant designs by changing the A constant which is determined by the lens thickness, lens form and lens location. It is derived by statistically analysing a series of patients retrospectively. Sanders and Kraff collaborated with Retzlaff [20] to subsequently set constants B and C at the same value for all implants and determined the best-fit A values for various implant types. The formula then became:

$$\text{IOL power} = A - 2.5 \times \text{axial length} - 0.9 \times \text{keratometry power}$$

This formula is commonly called the Sanders Retzlaff Kraff (SRK) formula. It may be personalized by the surgeon to account for the variability introduced by his surgical technique. The keeping of an accurate record of each IOL implantation allows an assessment of the error induced by the surgery and this can subsequently be incorporated into the A constant to improve the accuracy of the implant power prediction.

Axt [22] used a very similar formula to the above but included a value for the ACD which was subsequently found to be of no consequence, in that its incorporation did not improve the precision of the IOL power prediction to produce emmetropia. The Axt formula displayed a close correlation with the SRK formula and was used to draw up a table in order to simplify the approach to IOL power prediction. The table consists of columns of axial length measurements and rows of keratometer readings. This allows the IOL power to be deduced (to the nearest 0.50 D for the Sheet's IOL design). The formula can be used with other types of implant by adjusting the value of the A constant. The formula is, however, less accurate for patients with long axial lengths. Thompson et al. [23] derived a formula using polynomial regression analysis, in order to improve the accuracy of the IOL power calculation when the axial length is longer than 24.5 mm.

In fact there are two formulae as follows:

$$P = 63.162 - 0.854l - 0.0187l^2 + 0.261K - 0.0143K^2$$

for axial lengths greater than 24.5 mm, and

$$P = 131.94 - 2.78l - 1.10K$$

for axial lengths less than 24.5 mm. Where P = emmetropic IOL power; l = axial length

(mm); K = keratometer reading (mean k in dioptres) using the Haag Streit keratometer.

Regression analysis is only as accurate as the data from which the formula is derived. Thall et al. [24] used the regression formulae of Retzlaff [20], Sanders and Kraff [21] and Thompson et al. [23] to develop a PASCAL computer program which calculates the power of the IOL. The program also includes a term for the final refraction, if it is felt desirable to produce some residual myopia or hyperopia. Their program is designed to take the data base of a surgeon's results and compute the constants, A, B, C and D, in the equation which will then determine the IOL power for that individual surgeon.

The equation is of the form:

$$P = A - Bl - CK - DR$$

where P = IOL power; l = axial length (mm); K = keratometer reading (D); R = spherical equivalent postoperative refraction (D).

The increase in extracapsular operations has led to the original SKR formula being modified to a second generation formula (SKR 11) [25].

This is as follows:

$$P = A_1 - 0.9K - 2.5l$$

where P = power of IOL for emmetropia; Al = corrected A constant (see below); K = keratometer power reading; l = axial length.

Corrected A constant

If $l < 20$ mm, $A_1 = A + 3$.

If $l < 21$ but > 20 mm, $A_1 = A + 2$.

If $l < 22$ but > 21, then $A_1 = A + 1$.

If $l < 24.5$ but > 22 mm, $A_1 = A$.

If $l > 24.5$ mm then $A_1 = A - 0.5$.

The value of the uncorrected A constant depends on the type of IOL being used. Its value will be around 115.

Generally, all the formulae discussed above work well for average axial lengths. Some are more accurate predictors of IOL power for short eyes, while others are better for long eyes. If one formula is to be used, it may be better to use a regression formula that has been corrected to account for the individual surgeon bias and corrected to account for any unusual axial lengths, such as the SRK II.

10.9 The form of the IOL

A lot of attention has been given to the design of the IOL haptic to improve the physical stability of the lens in the eye and to reduce complications. However, little attention has been given to the optical design that may affect retinal image quality. IOLs are generally made in one of three simple forms:

(a) plano-convex with the curved surface facing the cornea;
(b) plano-convex with the curved surface facing the retina;
(c) biconvex.

Atchison [26] investigated the effect of the lens form on the optical performance of pseudophakic eyes. Image quality criteria included wave aberrations, spot diagrams, longitudinal aberrations, the modulation transfer function and an optimization procedure. He concluded that the optimum lens form for on-axis vision is close to the plano-convex form with the more curved surface facing the cornea. He believes that good IOL forms range from the plano-convex to the equi-convex. Plano-convex lenses with the curved surface facing the retina were found to be inferior.

10.10 Small-incision surgery

In the past, cataract surgery has required an arcuate corneal incision close to the limbus and about 7 mm in length. Sutures are used to close the wound which may induce 1.50 to 3.00 D of against-the-rule corneal astigmatism. This surgically induced astigmatism can be a nuisance, particularly when different amounts are present in the two eyes and/or the axes are oblique. This is not unusual and it can produce perceived distortion of three dimensional space. Small-incision surgery is revolutionizing this problem.

The surgeon makes an incision just outside the limbus which is about 3–4 mm long. An ultrasound probe is inserted through a hole in the anterior capsule to emulsify the lens within the capsular bag (phacoemulsification) and remove it by suction. New foldable implants made of silicone rubber (refractive index 1.43) are inserted through a tube, 3.5 mm in diameter, into the capsular bag. The implant centres well because it is surrounded by an intact capsular bag. Also, the small incision minimizes the problem of surgically induced astigmatism. It is probable that single suture or sutureless surgical wounds, pioneered in the late 80s, will see an end to surgically induced corneal astigmatism.

In the future, the possibility of bifocal or multifocal IOLs can be considered and there has been speculation concerning the viability of techniques where the contents of the capsule are removed and replaced with a fluid that mimics the lens substance, thus allowing the pseudophakic eye to accommodate.

References

1. Binkhorst, R.D. The optical design of intraocular lens implants. *Ophthalmic Surgery*, **6**, 17–31 (1975)
2. Binkhorst, R.D. Pitfalls in the determination of intraocular lens power without ultrasound. *Ophthalmic Surgery*, **7**, 69–73 (1976)
3. Hoffer, K. J. Preoperative cataract evaluation: Intraocular lens power calculation. *International Ophthalmology Clinic*, **22**, 37–75 (1982)
4. Strobel, J. and Jacobi, K.W. Posterior chamber lenses with convex side posteriorly – the calculation of dioptric power and results. *Transactions of the Ophthalmological Society of the UK*, **104**, 580–581 (1985)
5. Ossonig, K.C. Standardised echography: basic principles, clinical applications and results. *International Ophthalmology Clinic*, **19**, 127–210 (1979)
6. Binkhorst, R.D. Intraocular lens power calculation. *International Ophthalmology Clinic*, **19**, 237–252 (1979)
7. Longstaff, S. Factors affecting intraocular lens calculation. *Transactions of the Ophthalmological Society of the UK*, **105**, 642–646 (1986)
8. Hoffer, K.J. Accuracy of ultrasound in intraocular lens calculation. *Archives of Ophthalmology*, **99**, 1819–1823 (1981)
9. Richards, S.C. Clinical evaluation of six intraocular lens calculation formulas. *American Intraocular Implant Society Journal*, **11**, 153–158 (1985)
10. Katz, H.R. and Forster, R.K. Intraocular lens calculations in combined penetrating keratoplasty, cataract extraction and intraocular lens implantation. *Ophthalmology*, **92**, 1203–1207 (1985)
11. Binkhorst, C.D. and Loones, L.H. Intraocular lens power. *Transactions of the American Academy of Ophthalmology and Otolaringology*, **81**, 70–79 (1976)
12. Fyodorov, S.N., Linksz, A. and Galin, M.A. Calculation of the optical power of intraocular lenses. *Investigative Ophthalmology and Visual Science*, **14**, 625–628 (1975)
13. Fyodorov, S.N. and Kolinko, A.L. Estimation of optical power of the intraocular lens. *Vestnik Oftalmologic (Moscow)*, **57**, 735–740 (1967)
14. Colenbrander, M.C. Calculation of the power of an iris clip lens for distant vision. *British Journal of Ophthalmology*, **57**, 735–739 (1973)
15. Thijssen, J. M. The emmetropic and iseikonic implant lens: Computer calculation of the refractive power and its accuracy. *Ophthalmologica*, **171**, 467–486 (1975)

16. Fritz, K.J., Partamian, L.G., Leveille, A.S. and Kiernan, J.P. Intraocular lens power formulas. *Ophthalmology*, **88**, 432–433 (1981)

17. Hoffer, K.J. Intraocular lens calculation: The problem of the short eye. *Ophthalmic Surgery*, **12**, 269–272 (1981)

18. Shammas, H.J. The fudged formula for intraocular lens power calculations. *American Intraocular Implant Society Journal*, **8**, 350–352 (1982)

19. Loyd, T L. and Gills, J.P. Linear regression software for intraocular lens implant power calculation. *American Journal of Ophthalmology*, **102**, 405 (1986)

20. Retzlaff, J. A new intraocular lens calculation formula. *American Intraocular Implant Society Journal*, **6**, 148–152 (1980)

21. Sanders, D.R. and Kraff, M.C. Improvement of intraocular lens power calculation using empirical data. *American Intraocular Implant Society Journal*, **6**, 263–267 (1980)

22. Axt, J. Power calculations for the style-30 (Sheets Design) and other intraocular lenses. *CLAO Journal*, **9**, 102–106 (1983)

23. Thompson, J.T., Maumenee, E. and Baker, C.C. A new posterior chamber intraocular lens formula for axial myopes. *Ophthalmology*, **91**, 484–488 (1984)

24. Thall, E.H., Reinhart, W.J. and Sabol, D. Linear regression software for intraocular lens implant power calculation. *American Journal of Ophthalmology*, **101**, 597–599 (1986)

25. Sanders, D.R., Retzlaff, J. and Kraff, M.C. Comparison of the SRK 11 formula and other second generation formulas. *Journal of Cataract Refractive Surgery*, **14**, 136–141 (1988)

26. Atchison, D.A. Optical design of poly (methyl methacrylate) intraocular lenses. *Journal of Cataract Refractive Surgery*, **16**, 178–187 (1990)

11

The medical treatment of cataract

Sally A. Young

The medical and social implications of cataract are increasing with the demographic rise in the ageing population (see Chapter 1). The accumulated knowledge of the possible pathological mechanisms of cataractogenesis described in Chapters 2 and 3 has led to a rational programme of pharmacotherapeutic research into potential anticataract therapy, as opposed to surgical intervention.

The mechanisms that give the lens its characteristic optical properties are of particular interest. As described in Chapter 3, age-related cataract is accompanied by a decrease in low molecular weight soluble proteins [1] with a corresponding increase in insoluble proteins [2]. There is a high degree of evidence in favour of the hypothesis that lens opacification is linked to processes of protein denaturation, aggregation and precipitation.

This situation has favoured the development of rapidly expanding research into the pharmacological treatment and prevention of cataract by investigating the efficacy, pharmacology and toxicology of any agent capable of interfering with any one of the specific biochemical mechanisms of cataract formation.

11.1 Elimination of risk factors

Many investigators have described the development of cataract as being the result of multiple subthreshold cataractogenic stresses [3,4]. Each stress acting alone may be insufficient to cause cataract but a combination of the individual components can possibly cause cataract in some patients. It is possible that age is one of these cataractogenic stresses and that the superimposition of other toxic stresses on an ageing lens may accelerate the rate of cataract formation. This suggests that the elimination of one or more subcataractogenic stresses may delay or prevent further progression of the cataract. Any drug or agent with known cataractogenic properties should therefore be used as briefly, or at as low a dose, as possible.

Some of the more frequent clinically encountered toxic stresses are listed below:

(a) Corticosteroids. The use of topical and systemic corticosteroids is associated with the appearance of axial posterior subcapsular cataracts. Cataract development is dependent on both dose and duration. All patients requiring prolonged corticosteroid therapy should therefore be carefully evaluated with particular respect to the lens.

(b) Miotics. Prolonged use of miotics has been shown to be associated with the appearance of anterior subcapsular (ASC) vacuoles and opacities. Long-acting anticholinesterase agents used for the treatment of glaucoma were found to be a major risk factor for the development of cataract [5]. Use of these drugs has consequently declined.

(c) X-ray radiation. Exposure to ionizing radiation is associated with the development of posterior subcapsular (PSC) cataract, occurring 6–24 months later [6]. Neutron and alpha beams produce the greatest ionization and therefore the greatest risk of cataract formation. A small single dose of radiation may lead to the development of posterior opacities. Higher doses may result in progression of the cataract to involve the entire PSC zone. The importance of appropriate shielding of the lens must therefore be stressed.

(d) Ultraviolet (UV) radiation in sunlight. Exposure to UV radiation has been linked to increased nuclear brunescence. UV light of wavelength 320 to 400 nm is absorbed by the lens, producing a possible protective effect for the retina. Several studies have shown a positive association between the duration of exposure to sunlight and the prevalence of age-related cataract. Although there is, as yet, no proven evidence of UV damage to the lens, the routine addition of UV filters (blocking the transmission of wavelengths below 400 nm) to spectacle lenses may be a means of preventing cataract formation. The necessity of wearing protective filters on sun beds should also be stressed.

(e) Electricity. ASC, PSC and cortical cataracts may result from an electrical shock.

(f) Copper and iron. Intraocular foreign bodies containing copper may lead to the formation of 'sunflower' cataracts, the 'petals' extending towards the equator. Foreign bodies containing iron may result in brown ASC opacities, leading to significant loss of vision. Such cataracts are best prevented by immediate removal of the foreign body.

In conclusion, any drug or agent with known cataractogenic properties should be used with caution. Signs of development or progression of cataract should be noted at once by evaluation of the lens, both before and during treatment. Surgical intervention is considered when the cataractous change progresses far enough to interfere with the normal life style of the patient. A way to prevent the progression of the initial cataractous change would therefore be advantageous to the patient. Despite the fact that cataract is not a life-threatening condition and intraocular lens (IOL) implantation already exists as a reasonably satisfactory method of treatment, medical therapy is generally con-

sidered preferable to surgery, providing that it has some real benefit to the patient. Any anticataract agent must therefore be safe and relatively free from minor side-effects.

The following sections review the literature dealing with some of the more promising anticataract agents that have been investigated.

11.2 Anticataract agents

Numerous preparations have been marketed with claims of efficacy in preventing, delaying or even reversing cataracts. The rationale of the use of some agents has a scientific basis but few have had their efficacy well documented in properly controlled prospective clinical trials. Many agents even lack the benefit of valid preclinical evaluation. Any product claiming to reverse advanced cataractous changes should be discounted, since the drug would need to reverse irrevocable changes to the lens proteins.

The lens derives its nutrients solely from the aqueous humour through diffusion and various transport systems. Its metabolism is maintained primarily through anaerobic glycolysis. The lens uses the derived energy to sustain various transport systems and to maintain a high intracellular ratio of potassium to sodium. Cataracts are believed to result from either insult to the lens or from changes in biochemical parameters, which can lead to additional biochemical stress and subsequent opacity formation. These cataracts are accompanied by changes in biochemical parameters such as ion and nutrient levels, redox potential and metabolic output [7].

Many of the medical therapies for cataract are aimed at normalizing lens biochemistry [8]. The rationale for these products varies. Agents have been proposed to maintain the cellular electrolyte balance, to prevent oxidative insult to the cell membrane, or to supplement deficient nutritional factors. Since the lens is an avascular tissue, any substance administered topically to the eye, or given systemically, must reach the lens by diffusion through the aqueous humour. The ability of a substance to achieve an effective concentration in the aqueous is therefore an important factor in its efficacy and may dictate its route of administration [8].

Anticataract products under investigation include:

(a) aldose reductase inhibitors (ARIs), e.g. sorbinil;
(b) non-steroidal anti-inflammatory agents, e.g. aspirin and Bendazac lysine;
(c) sulphur-containing agents;
(d) inorganic salts;
(e) natural product extracts;
(f) vitamins.

11.2.1 Aldose reductase inhibitors

ARIs are generally considered to be among the most promising of agents for the medical treatment of cataract. Although none of the ARIs have been shown to delay cataract in man, such agents have been used successfully in animals to prevent galactosaemic and diabetic cataract formation. They have shown marked ability to prevent, or even normalize, some of the biochemical, functional and morphological changes that occur in other tissues containing the enzyme. These include the blood vessels of the kidney and retina, motor and sensory nerves and the cornea. The ARI sorbinil, for example, led to a reversible increase in motor nerve conduction velocity in 31 human diabetics [9]. This supports a role for the sorbitol pathway as a contributory factor in diabetic polyneuropathy. This has led to widespread optimism that such agents will be beneficial to human diabetics.

The process of sugar cataract development in experimental animal models is initiated by the adverse osmotic stress resulting from the intracellular accumulation of sorbitol, formed by the action of aldose reductase (AR). The inhibition of this enzyme could therefore represent a therapeutic approach by modifying the development of cataract in diabetes mellitus (DM). ARIs have been used both *in vitro* and *in vivo* [8] to inhibit the onset of cataract.

One of the most interesting properties of AR is that it attacks other aldehyde-containing compounds in addition to a variety of sugars [9]. There are many compounds that inhibit AR, probably because there are so many substrates for this enzyme. Early compounds, such as tetramethylene glutaric acid, were effective in preventing the synthesis and accumulation of polyol and vacuole formation in cultured lenses but were ineffective *in vivo*. Other compounds were unsuccessful because of low water solubility or inability to penetrate biological membranes. Natural products such as quercetin and rutoside were found to show ARI activity but failed because of their limited water solubility [10].

11.2.1.1 Fluorenone derivatives

An exciting breakthrough came with the development of the potent ARIs (AL 1567 and AL 1576). They were found to exhibit marked *in vitro* and *in vivo* efficacy against diabetic and galactosaemic cataracts, nerve conduction impairment and basement membrane thickening in retinal and renal capillaries [11]. Although highly potent in animal trials, the use of fluorenone derivatives in man is not possible at the present time because of adverse side effects.

11.2.1.2 Synthetic compounds

The most potent ARIs known are the synthetic compounds [12], the most widely tested of which is sorbinil. Sorbinil has been found to decrease the accumulation of sorbitol [13] and delay the onset of cataract in the diabetic rat [14]. The activity of sorbinil in the lens epithelium of the adult human was not as dramatic, however, with the human lens experiencing much less AR activity than the lens of the laboratory rat. Although the build up of sorbinil concentration in the human lens was found to be satisfactory [15], the drug was withdrawn from clinical trials because of its serious side-effects.

11.2.2 Non-steroidal anti-inflammatory drugs (NSAIDs)

Since most NSAIDs are organic acids, it is not surprising to find compounds reported to have anticataract activity within this class. Acetylsalicylic acid (aspirin) and Bendazac lysine are two such examples [7]. DeSantis [8] claims that both products also exhibit weak ARI activity (see Section 11.2.1). The two compounds are discussed below.

11.2.2.1 Aspirin

In 1981 it was reported that the prevalence of cataract was significantly lower in patients with rheumatoid arthritis on doses of 2.7 g aspirin per day for 10.4 years, compared with a matched population not receiving aspirin [16].

Diabetic patients receiving high doses of aspirin also appeared to show a decreased prevalence of cataracts [7]. These publications were criticized on the grounds of the classification of cataract severity by lens colour, a method that has not been validated [7].

Other publications suggested that aspirin decreases lens tryptophan. This is an amino acid that may be involved in lens pigmentation and brunescent cataract formation [17]. Lowered tryptophan levels supposedly reduce the risk of cataract. Elevated levels of both free and bound plasma tryptophan have been observed in patients with cataracts, aphakia and DM [18]. Free tryptophan and its metabolite kynurenine can be transported actively into lenses, where they accumulate and may bind to lens proteins. This has been observed with cultured lenses of rabbits and calves [19]. Reducing the available levels of tryptophan should therefore reduce the potential cataractogenic effects of elevated levels of tryptophan and kynurenine. Salicylic acid has been found to cause a release of bound tryptophan and a reduction in the total serum tryptophan concentration [20]. However, it was also reported that aspirin administration actually increases the concentration of free tryptophan by 50%. The increased levels of free tryptophan accumulated in the lens may then negate the anticataractogenic effect of the reduction in the total serum tryptophan concentration.

A group of workers from the National Eye Institute in the USA concluded that there was no overall beneficial effect of aspirin on either the occurrence or the rate of development of cataract. They concluded that evidence of a positive association between aspirin use and a lowered incidence of cataract was not adequate enough to justify a large-scale prospective clinical trial [6].

A number of recent clinical trials have been instigated to investigate the associations between aspirin use and cardiac disease and stroke. The Physicians' Health Survey [21], involving more than 20 000 American physicians taking aspirin or a placebo, investigated the use of aspirin as a preventative agent for myocardial infarction. A subset of this population was used to determine the prevalence of age-related cataract in the two populations. Aspirin was found to offer some protection against cataract development. A British trial of over 5000 male doctors found no significant

protection against myocardial infarction, stroke or cataract [22].

At present, the evidence supporting the use of aspirin as a means of preventing cataract is equivocal. Nevertheless, evidence from case control studies with large numbers of cataract patients appears to suggest that low doses of aspirin (together with paracetamol and ibuprofen) are associated with a halving of the risk of visually impairing lens opacities [23]. The risk of aspirin-related complications such as bleeding, gastric or duodenal ulceration and tinnitus are minimal when aspirin doses are low.

11.2.2.2 Bendazac lysine

Bendazac is a topical anti-inflammatory drug that inhibits some degenerative necrotic processes [24]. Bendazac L-lysine salt (1-benzyl-1H-indazol-3-yl-oxyacetic acid) was initially proposed as an NSAID [25]. Subsequently, it was observed that this compound exerted a highly antidenaturant effect on proteins and that it protected lens proteins against heat and X-rays [26]. It exhibited properties similar to those of other anti-inflammatory drugs (salicylate, oxyphenylbutazone, indomethacin, sulindac) which were found to inhibit lens and cataract AR [13]. Administration of this agent to galactosaemic rats has been reported to result in a delay in cataract formation, possibly as a result of its ability to inhibit AR [27]. It is currently available as an anticataract agent in Argentina, South Korea and several European countries. Clinical trials are now underway in the UK, Germany and Holland.

(a) In vitro *effects*

The antidenaturant activity of Bendazac has been studied in various types of protein denatured by different experimental techniques including, heat, UV rays and the addition of urea. Silvestrini *et al.* [25] found that Bendazac prevented changes in the turbidity induced by heating or by UV irradiation of different protein materials. It was also found to block the UV rays. Their results suggested that the blocking activity and the antidenaturant effects of Bendazac were two independent properties. The mode of action of Bendazac was described as the inhibition of heat-induced transformation of albumin but not of β- and γ-globulins. The binding of protein does not interfere with antidenaturant effects. Bendazac thus exerts a high degree of antidenaturant action on proteins. The effect is proportional to its absolute concentration, regardless of whether it is free or bound to proteins.

Musci and Silvestrini [28] investigated the mechanism of the scavenger-like activity of Bendazac. It has been reported that Bendazac inhibits the depolymerization of hyaluronic acid induced by $OH^{\bullet}$ or $O_2^{-\bullet}$ radicals, therefore implying that it is a free radical scavenger. This activity may contribute to the anticataract action of Bendazac. Musci and Silvestrini [28] further investigated the antidenaturant activity of Bendazac and suggested that it prevents albumin denaturation induced by urea, heat and free radicals. Their results indicated that Bendazac probably prevents both protease-mediated and free-radical-induced bovine serum albumin denaturation. Scavenger activity of Bendazac was not found where the target for free radicals was a substrate different from proteins. These results indicated that Bendazac is not a true scavenger but possesses a scavenger-like activity.

(b) In vivo *effects*

Despite the fact that the lens is an avascular organ with a poor biochemical exchange, Bendazac lysine salt has been found to have the capacity to exert effects similar to those observed *in vitro* following systemic treatment. Iuliano *et al.* [29] demonstrated that Bendazac lysine salt exerts a non-competitive inhibition of AR from the rat lens, which may provide an indication of Bendazac's anticataract potential.

It should be remembered, however, that tissue drug concentration may be crucial in determining clinical efficacy. Silvestrini *et al.* [30] demonstrated that, after a single oral administration in rats, the levels of Bendazac in the lens were very low compared with the serum levels. Some 24 h later, the concentration in the lens was found to have decreased by 33%. An oral dose of Bendazac to inhibit AR would therefore need to be very high and could induce side effects. Ballestreros *et al.* [31] reported two cases of hepatitis in patients receiving oral Bendazac lysine salt. It would seem that such difficulties could be resolved by using eye drops with the appropriate drug concentration. Although Silvestrini *et al.* [25] recommended topical administration of Bendazac, having demonstrated its high corneal permeability, poor topical efficacy has been noted by all subsequent workers.

(c) *Clinical trials in man*

After satisfactory safety and tolerance tests had taken place in man, the first study on the anticataract activity of Bendazac was performed at the University of Naples Eye Clinic [32]. The study included 17 patients with age-related cataract, each with a medical history of rapid increase in grade of opacification. The patients were aged between 47 and 73 years and 0.5 g of Bendazac was administered three times daily at meal times. The mean duration of treatment was 72 days. No side effects were reported during the course of treatment. The authors claimed a decrease in lens opacity in 22 eyes, no change in six eyes and deterioration in one eye. A significant improvement in VA was also found. The degree of improvement was thought to depend on the extent and morphology of the cataract, with early and cortical opacities responding better to treatment.

Bendazac was compared with placebo in a double-blind controlled multicentre study [33] of 80 patients with age-related cataract. Refractive error, visual acuity (VA) and slit-lamp lens evaluation were performed at baseline, after 1 month and after the 3 month endpoint. VA was found to improve significantly in the Bendazac group and deteriorate significantly in the placebo group. Assessment of change in lens opacities showed a decrease in 12 out of 47 eyes in the Bendazac group, as compared with three out of 40 eyes in the placebo group.

A similar study by Testa *et al.* [34] was performed on 40 patients affected with age-related cataract and a general tendency towards rapid deterioration. A daily intake of 1.5 g of Bendazac was prescribed for a 3-month period. At the end of the study, no improvement was found in the placebo-treated group but a progressive improvement in VA was noted in the Bendazac-treated group.

A number of open studies have also been carried out [33,35–40]. The average duration of treatment for the combined studies was 6.8 months (ranging from 1 month to 11 months). In a total of 413 eyes, VA was unchanged in 60.3%, improved in 36.8% and worsened in 2.9% of cases. Slit-lamp lens opacity evaluation showed no change in 72.4%, improvement in 26.5% and deterioration in 1.1% of cases.

Tolerance was generally found to be good in all studies. For the combined open studies, adverse side-effects (mainly gastrointestinal disturbances) were reported in 8.4% of cases.

Criticism has been associated with the use of uncontrolled open studies and the over-reliance on VA as a measure of cataract progression. Hockwin *et al.* [41] used densitometric scanning of Scheimpflug slit image photographs to assess the degree of light scatter by the lens in a placebo-controlled double-blind clinical trial over an 18-month period. No differences between the two groups were noted when the cataract morphologies were combined for assessment. There was a possible improvement in cortical and nuclear opacities in the Bendazac-treated group.

11.2.3 Redox/sulphur-containing agents and free radical scavengers

A number of sulphur-containing reducing agents are available as anticataract formulations. Anticataract action arises from the oxidation of some of the many sulphydryl components in the lens, which are a feature of cataract.

As described in Chapter 2, there is a loss of reduced glutathione from the lens during cataract formation. Glutathione may protect various sulphydryl components in the lens through its ability to serve as a reducing agent. In diabetic animals treated with the fluorenone derivatives AL 1567 and AL 1576 (see Section 11.2.1.1), glutathione levels are maintained in the normal range [42]. DeSantis [8] speculates that lenticular levels of NADPH, a reduced form of the coenzyme NAD, may be too low to allow sufficient reduction of the oxidized glutathione to occur. This is possibly due to excessive AR activity in periods of high cellular glucose. In addition, oxidized glutathione may leak from the cell and contribute to depletion of cellular reduced glutathione. When AR activity is inhibited, NADPH levels are possibly sufficient to maintain activity of the enzyme glutathione reductase.

Although reduced glutathione can be actively incorporated into the lens, lenticular glutathione levels are maintained through rapid synthesis from its constituent amino acids rather than from specific transport [43]. Preparations containing the three constituent amino acids of glutathione (glutamic acid, glycine and cysteine) have therefore been formulated to increase the lenticular levels of glutathione. Kern and Ho [44], however, reported that, in specific transport studies of the bovine lens, little of the glutamic acid does, in fact, enter the lens. Clinical studies have shown only slight, if any, changes in patients with early cataracts treated in this way [45].

Superoxide dismutase, an enzyme that acts as a scavenger of the superoxide radical, is also used as an anticataract agent [46].

11.2.4 Inorganic salts

A simple approach to cataract therapy has been the use of inorganic salts intended as a substitute for, or supplement to, inorganic lens constituents, or to produce dehydration of the lens by an osmotic action. Formulations typically contain strontium salts (iodide, iodate, chloride and nitrate), calcium, potassium and sodium. Agents are applied as eye drops. Some products combine one or more inorganic salt with a nutritional substance, usually a vitamin (Section 11.2.6) or a natural product extract (Section 11.2.5) [7].

11.2.5 Natural product extracts

Various preparations contain extracts of natural products of plant or animal origin. Examples are digitalis, digitoxin and plant extracts from *Hamamelis vulgaris* (witch hazel) [7]. Some preparations combine vitamin iodide/iodate formulations with glycosides such as digitoxin or digitalis. These agents can alter the aqueous flow through their apparent ability to inhibit the enzyme Na^+,K^+-ATPase [47]. Although these cardiac glycosides are also potentially cataractogenic, as a result of their ability to inhibit lens Na^+,K^+-ATPase, cataracts are not associated with them because of their low distribution in the lens [48].

Products of animal origin include glandular extracts from thyroid, parathyroid, ovaries and testes [7]. In some formulations, animal extracts are combined with vitamins, minerals and iodide/iodate salts.

The use of hormones or crude organ extracts is questionable, since the relationship between endocrine dysfunction and cataract is not significant. Kuck [49] suggests that none of the target glands of the pituitary (which include the thyroid, ovaries and testes) significantly control lens growth.

11.2.6 Vitamins

Although nutritional factors may play a role in determining the rate of cataract formation, or susceptibility of the lens to other damaging agents, there is no firm evidence that nutritional deficiencies, as such, cause opacification [50].

One current viewpoint is that the symptoms of diarrhoea may play a role in cataractogenesis [23]. Diarrhoea co-exists with malnutrition in many Third World nations where cataract is prevalent. The theory identifies at least four effects of the diarrhoea syndrome that may affect the lens:

(a) malabsorption of nutrients including fats, carbohydrates, amino acids and vitamins;
(b) systemic acidosis;
(c) dehydration with associated osmotic imbalances and electrolyte disturbances;
(d) increased blood urea with subsequent osmotic effects, disruption of proteins or carbamylate amino acids and reaction with thiol groups [23].

As with DM or hyperglycaemia, diarrhoea and/ or its consequences might be causative of cataract, or act as contributing/predisposing factors.

There are many anticataract products containing vitamins. Some are simple combinations of vitamins, while others combine vitamins with minerals, hormones and other natural products [7]. There are a number of B vitamins in anticataract products, with thiamine (B_1), riboflavin (B_2), nicotinamide (B_3), pantothenic acid (B_5) and pyridoxine (B_6) all being used [7]. The use of B vitamins appears to be based on their involvement as enzyme cofactors.

The biochemical function of retinol (vitamin A) in the lens is unknown, although it has been associated with the maintenance of membranes and protein synthesis in other tissues.

Other vitamins, particularly vitamins C and E, act as antioxidants against oxidative substances that have been shown to cause cataractous changes. The hydrophilic ascorbic acid (vitamin C) does not readily penetrate the cornea. It is, however, actively secreted into the aqueous humour by the ciliary processes and can achieve a relatively high concentration in the eye when given systemically. Vitamin C has been shown to serve as a free scavenger and antioxidant in the lens [51].

The principal anticataract function of vitamin E (a lipid-soluble antioxidant) is believed to be protection of lipid membranes from free-radical attack. Scanning electron microscopy has been used to show that vitamin E (or mixtures of vitamin E with glutathione) can have a protective effect against cortical cataracts in rats [52–54].

11.3 Conclusions

Most clinicians are in agreement that no medical treatment of cataract, other than surgery, currently exists [7]. Anticataract agents are prescribed to patients, however, as a placebo to reassure them that treatment is taking place before cataract surgery. Medical therapy would nevertheless be an attractive form of treatment, if it could inhibit the progression of a lens opacity or even restore its original transparency.

As medical intervention becomes a possibility, the demand will increase for objective methods of documenting the changes associated with cataract. The measurement of VA alone is not an accurate enough clinical evaluation of the progression of cataract. Composite protocols (including various combinations of photographic, structural and functional measurements) must therefore be employed in the careful evaluation of a potential anticataract agent. Cataract development is most probably triggered by a multitude of factors. At present, only AR involvement in sugar cataract formation has been identified as a formative mechanism in man. Potent ARIs therefore represent the most promising anticataract agents currently under development.

References

1. Francois, J., Rabaey, M. and Stockmans, S.L. Gel filtration of the soluble proteins from normal and cataractous human lenses. *Experimental Eye Research,* **4**, 312–318 (1965)
2. Croft, L.R. Low molecular weight proteins of the lens. In *The Human Lens in Relation to Cataract; Ciba Foundation Symposium,* 19, Elsevier, Excerpta Medica, Amsterdam, pp. 207–224 (1973)
3. Hiller, R., Sperduto, R.D. and Ederer, F. Epidemiologic associations with nuclear, cortical and posterior subcapsular cataract. *American Journal of Epidemiology,* **124**, 916–925 (1986)
4. Harding, J.J. and van Heyningen, R. Case-control study of cataract in Oxford. *Developments in Ophthalmology,* **15**, 99–103 (1987)
5. Pirie, A. Chairman's concluding remarks. *Ciba Foundation Symposium,* **19**, 311–313 (1973)
6. Chylack, L.T. The crystalline lens and cataract. In *Manual of Ocular Diagnosis and Therapy* (edited by D. Pavan-

Langston), Little, Brown and Company, Boston/Toronto, pp. 117–138 (1985)

7. Kador, P. Overview of the current attempts toward the medical treatment of cataract. *Ophthalmology,* **90,** 352–364 (1983)

8. DeSantis, L. New horizons in the medical therapy of cataract: aldose reductase inhibitors and other agents. *Pharmacy International,* 17–20 (1986)

9. Kinoshita, J.H., Kador, P.F. and Catiles, M. Aldose reductase in diabetic cataracts. *JAMA,* **246,** 257–261 (1981)

10. Varma, S.D. and Kinoshita, J.H. *Biochemical Pharmacology,* **25,** 2505–2513 (1976)

11. Chandler, M.L., Shannon, W.A. and DeSantis, L. *Investigative Ophthalmology and Visual Science,* **25** (Supplement), 159 (1984)

12. Kador, P.F., Robison, W.G. and Kinoshita, J.H. *Annual Review of Pharmacology and Toxicology,* **25,** 691–714 (1985)

13. Sharma, Y.R. and Cotlier, E. Inhibition of lens and cataract aldose reductase by protein-bound antirheumatic drugs: salicylate, indomethacin, oxyphenbutazone, sulindac. *Experimental Eye Research,* **35,** 21–27 (1982)

14. Fukuski, S., Merola, L.O. and Kinoshita, J.H. Altering the course of cataracts in diabetic rats. *Investigative Ophthalmology and Visual Science,* **19,** 313–315 (1980)

15. Crabbe, M.J.C. Partial sequence homology of human myc oncogene protein to beta and gamma crystallins. *FEBS Letters,* **181,** 157–159 (1985)

16. Cotlier, E. and Sharma, Y.R. Aspirin and senile cataracts in rheumatoid arthritis. *Lancet,* **1,** 338–339 (1981)

17. Zigler, J.S. Jr and Goosey, J.D. Photosensitized oxidation in the ocular lens. Evidence for photosensitizers endogenous to the human lens. *Photochemistry and Photobiology,* **33,** 869–974 (1981)

18. Cotlier, E., Sharma, Y.R. and Zuckerman, J. Plasma tryptophan in humans with diabetic and senile cataracts. *Experimental Eye Research,* **33,** 247–252 (1981)

19. Schweitzer, J. and Cotlier, E. Kynurenine: active transport by crystalline lens. *ARVO Abstracts. Investigative Ophthalmology and Visual Science,* **19** (Supplement), 265 (1980)

20. Smith, H.G. and Lakatos, C. Effects of acetylsalicylic acid on serum protein binding and metabolism of tryptophan in man. *Journal of Pharmacy and Pharmacology,* **23,** 180–189 (1971)

21. Physicians' Health Study Research Group. Preliminary report: findings from the aspirin component of the ongoing Physicians' Health Study. *New England Journal of Medicine,* **318,** 262–264 (1988)

22. Peto, R., Gray, R., Collins, R. *et al.* Randomised trial of prophylactic daily aspirin in British male doctors. *British Medical Journal,* **296,** 313–316 (1988)

23. Harding, J.J. In *Molecular and Cellular Biology of the Eye Lens* (edited by H. Bloemendal), Wiley and Sons, New York, pp. 327–365 (1981)

24. Silvestrini, B. Rationale for bendazac. In *Recent Developments in the Pharmacological Treatment of Cataract* (edited by F. D'Ermo, F. Ponte and A.M. Laties), Kugler Publications, Amsterdam, pp. 1–9 (1987)

25. Silvestrini, B., Catanese, B., Lisciani, R. and Alessandroni, A. Studies on the mechanism of action of bendazac (AF 983). *Drug Research,* **20,** 250–253 (1970)

26. Pandolfo, L., Livrea, M.A. and Bono, A. Effects of bendazac-L-lysine salt on X-ray-induced cataract in the rabbit lens. *Experimental Eye Research,* **42,** 167–175 (1986)

27. Iuliano, G., Colapinto, F., Santino, D. and Libondi, T. Effetto protettivo dell 1-benzil-3-indazol-ossiacetato nelia cataratta galattosemica sperimentale del ratto. In *Bendazac L-Lysine Salt: Investigators' Brochure,* F. Angelini Research Institute, Rome (1984)

28. Musci, G. and Silvestrini, B. Mechanism of the scavenger-like activity of bendazac. *Drugs in Experimental Clinical Research,* **13,** 289–292 (1987)

29. Iuliano, G., Menzione, M., Apponi-Battini, G. and Costagliola, C. Inhibition of rat lens aldose reductase by Bendazac-L-lysine salt. *Enzyme,* **42,** 235–237 (1989)

30. Silvestrini, B., Catanese, B., Barillari, G., Iorio, E. and Valerui, P. Basic data supporting the use of L-lysine salt of bendazac in cataract. In *Recent Developments in the Pharmacological Treatment of Cataract* (edited by F. D'Ermo, F. Ponte and A.M. Laties), Kugler Publications, Amsterdam (1987)

31. Ballestreros, J.A., Badosa, A.M., Usandizaga, I. and Amengual, M. Hepatoxicity due to bendazac. *Lancet,* **ii,** 1030–1031 (1987)

32. Testa, M., Iuliano, G. and Silvestrini, B. Pilot study of bendazac for treatment of cataract. *Lancet,* **1,** 849–850 (1982)

33. Mannucci, L.L., Doro, D. and Angi, M.R. Valutazione clinica del bendazac-lisina nella terapia della cataratta presenile e senile. In *Bendazac L-Lysine Salt: Investigators' Brochure,* F. Angelini Research Institute, Rome (1984)

34. Testa, M., Iuliano, G., De Gregorio, M. and Pioggia, M. A double-blind clinical study on the anticataract effect of bendazac lysine salt. *Acta Therapeutica,* **9,** 235–252 (1983)

35. Leoni, R. and Baroncini, R. Esperienze con bendalina nella terapia della cataratta. Minerva Oftalmologica, 24, 1-12 (1982). In *Bendazac L-Lysine Salt: Investigators' Brochure,* F. Angelini Research Institute, Rome (1984)

36. Boschi, G., Casacci, M. and Lia, A. L'uso del bendazac lisina – bendaline – nella terapia della cataratta. Minerva Oftalmologica 24, 1–7 (1982). In *Bendazac L-Lysine Salt: Investigators' Brochure,* F. Angelini Research Institute, Rome (1984)

37. Calogero, R., Moro, A. and Della Costa, L. Bendazac lisina nella terapia della cataratta. In *Bendazac L-Lysine Salt: Investigators' Brochure,* F. Angelini Research

Institute, Rome (1984)

38. Merlin, V., Rivieri, G.B., Boandini, M. and Pareschi, A. Sui risultati della sperimentazione terapeutica nella cataratta senile con bendazac sale di lisina – bendalina. In *Bendazac L-Lysine Salt: Investigators' Brochure*, F. Angelini Research Institute, Rome (1984)

39. Testa, M., Iuliano, G., DeGregorio, M. and Pioggia, M. A controlled clinical study on bendazac lysine salt treatment in senile cataract. *Acta Therapeutica*, **10**, 35–48 (1984). In *Bendazac L-Lysine Salt: Investigators' Brochure*, F. Angelini Research Institute, Rome (1984)

40. Gallo, O. and DeRosa, G. Valutazione clinica sull impiego della bendalina in pazienti affetti da cataratta. In *Bendazac L-Lysine Salt: Investigators' Brochure*, F. Angelini Research Institute, Rome (1984)

41. Hockwin, O., Laser, H., DeGregorio, M. and Carrieri, M.P. Bendazac lysine in selected types of human senile cataract. *Ophthalmic Research*, **21**, 141–154 (1989)

42. York, B., Lou, M., Chyan, O. and Chandler, M.L. *Investigative Ophthalmology and Visual Science*, **26** (Supplement), 303 (1985)

43. Reddy, V.N., Varma, S.D. and Chakrapani, B. Transport and metabolism of glutathione in the lens. *Experimental Eye Research*, **16**, 105–114 (1973)

44. Kern, H.L. and Ho, C.K. Transport of L-glutamic acid and L-glutamine and their incorporation into lenticular glutathione. *Experimental Eye Research*, **17**, 455–462 (1973)

45. Hockwin, O., Kietzmann, M.T., Vanar-Matiar, H. and Edeibi, A. Concentration of glutamic acid, glycine and cysteine in the aqueous humour of rabbits after topical and peroral application. *Ophthalmic Research*, **10**, 250–258 (1978)

46. Hockwin, O. and Koch, H.R. In *Cataract and Abnormalities of the Lens* (edited by J.G. Bellows), Grune and Stratton, New York, pp. 243–254 (1974)

47. March, W.F., Goren, S.B. and Shoch, D. Cardioactive glycosides in ophthalmology. In *Symposium on Ocular Therapy* (edited by I.H. Leopold), CV Mosby, St. Louis, vol. 6, pp. 11–18 (1973)

48. Lufkin, M.W., Harrison, C.E. Jr, Henderson, J.W. and Ogle, K.N. Ocular distribution of digoxin-3H in the cat. *American Journal of Ophthalmology*, **64**, 1134–1140 (1967)

49. Kuck, J.F.R. Jr. Metabolism of the lens. In *Biochemistry of the Eye* (edited by C.N. Graymore), Academic Press, New York, pp. 307–312 (1970)

50. Bunce, G.E. Nutrition and cataract. *Nutrition Reviews*, **37**, 337–343 (1979)

51. Kuck, J.F.R. Jr. Composition of the lens. In *Cataract and Abnormalities of the Lens* (edited by J.G. Bellows), Grune and Stratton, New York, pp. 69–96 (1975)

52. Creighton, M.O., Sanwal, M. and Trevithick, J.R. In vitro modelling and prevention of steroid cataract. *ARVO Abstracts. Investigative Ophthalmology and Visual Science*, **20**, 127 (1981)

53. Stewart-DeHan, P.J., Creighton, M.O., Sanwal, M. *et al.* Effects of vitamin E on cortical cataractogenesis induced by elevated temperature in intact rat lenses in medium 199. *Experimental Eye Research*, **32**, 51–60 (1981)

54. Trevithick, J.R., Ross, W.M., Creighton, M.O. and Sanwals, M. Comparison of galactose and glucose induced cataractogenesis and preventative effects of vitamin E *in vitro* and *in vivo*. *ARVO Abstracts. Investigative Ophthalmology and Visual Science*, **20** (Supplement), 219 (1981)

Index

Printed and bound by CPI Group (UK) Ltd, Croydon, CR0 4YY

08/05/2025

01864767-0001